Fountain of Health

Regain Your Health, Happiness, and Lose Weight. A Revolution in Health for Everybody

Manuel Moran, M.D., Ph.D., J.D.

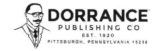

DORRANCE
PUBLISHING CO
EST. 1920
PITTSBURGH, PENNSYLVANIA 15238

Dorrance Publishing Co
585 Alpha Drive
Suite 103
Pittsburgh, PA 15238
Visit our website at *www.dorrancebookstore.com*

ISBN: 978-1-6491-3107-2
eISBN: 978-1-6491-3614-5

PREVENTION, PREVENTION, PREVENTION is the key concept. It is much easier and inexpensive to remain healthy than to reverse chronic medical conditions. Growing old is unavoidable at this time, with "modern" technology, but chronic pains and diseases are preventable. Take action while you are still symptoms-free. Well-established cancers are difficult to treat and frequently are not curable by modern medicine. A significant percentage of patients die from the treatment (e.g., complications from chemotherapy).

Are you willing to take action to remain healthy and happy or are you going to suffer the wrath of chronic degenerative diseases, cancer, and obesity? Believe it or not, your wellbeing is in your hands.

These guidelines will help weight control and usually will prevent or decrease/reverse cardiovascular disease (heart attacks, strokes, etc.) as well as many cancers and other chronic degenerative diseases like osteoarthritis, hypertension, type 2 diabetes, autoimmune diseases, autism, attention deficit disorder, dementia/Alzheimer's disease, other mental or behavioral conditions in children or teenagers, ovarian polycystic disease (which causes infertility), erectile dysfunction, etc. In general, no need to count calories or to attempt to reduce your total calorie intake.

The reader is advised to read the books *Fat for Fuel* by Dr. Joseph Mercola and *The Plant Paradox* by Dr. Steven Gundry. The web page www.mercola.com has very extensive health information. For type 2 diabetics you will benefit from reading *How Not to Die* by Dr. Michael Greger and *Reversing Diabetes* by Dr. Neal D. Barnard.

Should the ideal diet be low fat or high fat, low carbohydrates or high carbohydrates, and so on? Much more important than the macronutrient percentages (fat, protein, carbohydrates) is the quality of the food ingested. Some conditions benefit from specific ratios (e.g., a ketogenic diet is good for children with epilepsy, weight loss, and cancer therapy). The same principle applies to other misused labels, like vegan, vegetarian, etc. A vegan eating Oreo cookies, as shown in a Netflix documentary, will not do well. An ideal diet will have small blood glucose (blood sugar) spikes and will keep fasting insulin levels low. For people without type 2 diabetes the IDEAL DIET is a mostly plant-based ORGANIC diet, that is:

- High in healthy fats that have been not heated or not heated to high temperatures. No unhealthy fats (no exceptions).
- No refined carbohydrates. No grains. No sugar.
- No processed foods.
- Normal or low protein for adults. Somewhat higher protein for children, athletes, and persons older than age 65.

With type 2 diabetes the ideal diet is all plant-based without animal fat, low in fat, and avoids excess calories. This diet will also improve neuropathy (nerve pain) symptoms.

Forget about the now obsolete "food pyramid" with grains at the bottom. Big financial interests are at stake but are beyond the scope if this review. Have you ever considered why healthy organic vegetables are not subsidized? Why subsidies go to food products scientifically proven to be unhealthy? What would be the actual cost of a cheeseburger at a fast food restaurant if the food industry was not subsidized?

Heart attacks (myocardial infarctions) are caused by coronary artery disease (calcification, plaque, narrowing or blockage with acute blood clots). It is often referred to as heart disease and these guidelines will use this term accordingly.

It would be ideal to keep a normal BMI (body mass index) of 18.5 to 24.9. Nevertheless, several factors like increased muscle volume affect the health predictive value of BMI. A more accurate indicator for some people is to measure the abdominal (belly) circumference at the level of the umbilicus (belly button) and divided it by height. It should be less than 0.5.

NO TOBACCO. Needless to say, no smoking or tobacco products. If you quit smoking, make sure you do not gain extra weight and become obese in the process.

INTRODUCTION

IT IS DIFFICULT, IF NOT IMPOSSIBLE, for the average citizen to understand how we got to this epidemic of chronic degenerative conditions in the USA, including heart attacks, strokes, diabetes, hypertension (high blood pressure), autoimmune diseases, cancers, autism, dementia, osteoarthritis, etc. In fact, many people wrongly assume this is part of normal aging. The risk of getting a cancer was one in three recently but some experts have revised it to one in two persons. Cancers were rare in the beginning of the 20th century. About two thirds of our population is obese or overweight, with other Western countries following closely. About half of the USA population has prediabetes or type 2 diabetes, a very expensive and devastating disease that now also affects children and teenagers, something that was unheard of just a few decades ago. About two thirds of people have hypertension by age 60. Autism has skyrocketed from 1 in 10,000 several decades ago to about in 60. "About 1 in 59 children has been identified with autism spectrum disorder" based on CDC data. [1] Interestingly, autism prevalence still remains very low in the Amish community although this is not a surprise. The number of patients suffering from dementia continues rising. It is already the most expensive disease affecting 37.4 percent of those age 90 or older [2]. Alzheimer is the most frequent type of dementia. It affects 5.8 million Americans in the USA, and this number is expected to increase to nearly 14 million by 2050. By then it is expected to cost the nation $1.1 trillion. [3]

This epidemic of chronic diseases seems to have no end in sight, as it keeps getting worse every year. Sooner or later it will bankrupt the nation. Either some healthcare will not be available or it will have to be significantly rationed…

---

1   https://www.cdc.gov/ncbddd/autism/data.html (accessed on 3-17-2019)

2   https://www.ncbi.nlm.nih.gov/pmc/articles/PMC2705925/ (accessed on 3-17-2019)

3   (https://www.alz.org/alzheimers-dementia/facts-figures (accessed on 3-17-2019)

unless appropriate measures are taken. You do not believe me? Dr. Mark Hyman wrote in Dr. Tom O'Bryan's book *The Autoimmune Fix* "by the year 2030 close to half of the population will be diagnosed with some form of chronic disease" and "it's predicted that by 2044 the cost of Medicare and Medicaid to treat these chronic conditions will be more than all the taxes collected by our government."

The incentive for the healthcare industry in general and for the pharmaceutical industry in particular is to treat, NOT to prevent chronic conditions. The financial incentive is not in preventing chronic conditions with simple dietary changes and other lifestyle changes. Taking a diabetes medication for life is much more profitable for the pharmaceutical industry than preventing the onset of diabetes. The same principle is applicable to the profit-geared food industry, which focuses on "convenient food" disregarding how inconvenient and expensive it is when people eating their food products develop chronic medical problems or cancer. To understand how we got here, the reader is encourage reading G. Edward Griffin's book *World Without Cancer*.

In the middle of this chaotic picture there is a ray of hope. In fact, 70 to 90 percent of all chronic degenerative conditions can be prevented following simple common sense guidelines. Prevention, not treatment, is the key word here. Your health is in your hands. A doctor with knowledge in these issues should be able to assist you and order the appropriate work up.

SUMMARY

1. RECOMMENDATIONS FOR FOOD AND COOKING.

1.1. AVOID PROCESSED FOODS.

This is THE MOST important change you can make.

1.2. EAT GOOD FATS BUT AVOID ALL BAD FATS.

This is CRITICAL to remain healthy. Bad fats are much worse to your health than tobacco. NO EXCEPTIONS to this recommendation. Unhealthy fats include all man-made fats (e.g., trans fats or partially hydrogenated oils, inter-esterified fats, margarines, Crisco), all processed vegetable oils (e.g., canola, corn, cottonseed, safflower, sunflower, soybean), and ALL healthy oils that have been exposed to high temperatures (or maybe even medium temperatures). Stay away from peanut oil, also. Buy organic oils and fats, thus NON-GMO (genetically modified organism or food) products. Do not buy any grain-fed fat because it has too many omega 6 fatty acids, in addition to other problems. Acceptable oils include extra virgin olive oil, cold pressed avocado oil, and organic coconut oil. Flax seed oil is healthy but unstable and should be stored in the refrigerator. All raw, unroasted nuts are healthy except for cashews (contain lectins) and peanuts (are not nuts but legumes). Grass-fed lard, butter, and saturated animal fats are acceptable in moderation as long as you do not have prediabetes or type 2 diabetes. But do not eat them if the animal has been grain-fed. And do not eat extra amounts just because saturated fats do not cause heart disease because they are pro-inflammatory and increase the risk of type 2 diabetes. Fats in general, and even more fish oil, decrease appetite and help weight loss.

1.3. AVOID, OR AT LEAST MINIMIZE, EATING OUT AT RESTAURANTS.

Most restaurant cook with unhealthy oils (processed vegetable oils) and/or at high temperatures. Many—if not most—reuse cooking vegetable oils time after time, which is a very harmful practice because every time the oil is heated it becomes more harmful. You should not routinely eat at restaurants in general and much less at fast food restaurants. If you eat out, do it only as an exception for special occasions and go to a higher-end restaurant that offers healthy choices.

1.4. DO NOT EAT ANY SUGAR OR ANY REFINED CARBOHYDRATES.

Refined carbohydrates (standing alone) do not exist in nature and are quite harmful to your health. They greatly increase the risk of heart attacks which are still the leading cause of early deaths. Sugar and refined carbohydrates are pro-inflammatory and decrease your body's pH (same thing happens with too much animal protein). Chronic inflammation is the root of all chronic conditions, including heart attacks and cancer. By lowering the body's pH, cancer cells and viruses will grow more easily. The body will try to buffer the pH by "robbing" precious minerals from the bones, thus leading to osteoporosis. Sugar and refined carbohydrates cause obesity and also have been linked to type 2 diabetes (even though they are not the actual cause of diabetes).

In addition, sugar and refined carbohydrates are nutrient depleted. It is difficult enough getting all necessary nutrients while eating a healthy diet, and it would be almost impossible when eating nutrient depleted foods. The food industry statement "a calorie is a calorie" when talking about weight control and calorie intake is totally incorrect (I am being polite by avoiding the word "lie") from a metabolic point of view because the way different foods are metabolized and used by the body.

Sugar creates a very strong addiction, difficult but not impossible to cure.

1.5. MINIMIZE FRUCTOSE

Fructose (sugar is half fructose) is a metabolic poison which in larger amounts causes fatty liver disease, hepatic (liver) insulin resistance (which increases the risk of diabetes), and obesity among other conditions. It is found in fruits but the food industry loves it because high fructose corn syrup is inexpensive. Do not buy any foods with added sugar or fructose. Avoid all fruit juices even the so-called "natural". Eating one or two pieces of fruit per is day acceptable, and you may add a reasonable number of berries, like blueberries.

1.6. DO NOT EAT ANY GLUTEN AND AVOID ALL GRAINS.

Gluten is a neurotoxin (damages nerves), and it should be COMPLETELY AVOIDED. Besides being a contributor to dementia, gluten will cause ataxia (unstable gate, falls) because it damages the cerebellum. It takes about 5 decades for the neurotoxic effect to start showing up. Once nerve damage has occurred, though, it is irreversible.

Gluten stimulates appetite and increases daily calorie intake by several hundred calories (about 400 calories/day) because it stimulates certain brain centers. This has been known for many decades.

Gluten causes a leaky gut, which increases chronic inflammation and many auto-immune conditions.

Avoid all grains because they have unhealthy lectins (a type of protein plants have to protect themselves), even the so called "healthy" grains like quinoa. Lectins in grains cannot be destroyed by pressure cooking.

Gluten has "morphine like" properties, so it will take some effort to get over the cravings.

A possible exception is ancient wheat, like Einkorn, if eaten in moderation or very small amounts. Einkorn only has 14 chromosomes compared to 42 for modern wheat, and thus has less gluten. We do not know whether Einkorn will cause nerve damage in the long run. No long-term studies have been preformed. Nevertheless, at least one study found gut mucosal damage (leaky gut) when animals were fed modern gluten but none when they were fed Einkorn. Einkorn is in the avoid list of food products from Dr. Stephen Gundry. Eat Einkorn at your own risk.

1.7. CONSUME ORGANIC FOODS.

This is VERY IMPORTANT. Long-term it is not more expensive. In fact, it will save you money in medical care and bills as well as quite a bit of physical and emotional suffering in the long run. AVOID ALL GMO (genetically modified organism) foods. Most come with glyphosate (the main ingredient in Round Up®, a herbicide) and other pesticides which are harmful to your health. In addition, genetically modified foods have less nutritional value.

1.8. EAT MOSTLY A PLANT-BASED DIET.

Eat whole foods prepared or cooked at home. Only 10 to 15 percent of calories should be from animal products. An ideal diet for persons WITHOUT prediabetes or type 2 diabetes is high in healthy plant-based fats (ideally not heated), no bad fats, normal/low protein (only whatever your needs are), no refined or simple carbohydrates, and carbohydrates but only those found in whole foods. This diet should be mostly vegetables, some healthy fruits, many raw nuts, and some pressure-cooked legumes if you are not sensitive to them.

Although saturated fats from grass-fed or free-range animals do not increase the risk of heart disease, they significantly increase the risk for type 2 diabetes. Again, DO NOT EAT any grain-fed animal products. Excess animal protein increases cancer risk. Red meat increases cancers more than other animal products due to a specific protein found in red meat.

FRESH food is much better if you have a choice. Avoid as much as possible canned or frozen products. Free-range eggs in moderation are acceptable but avoid them if you have prediabetes or type 2 diabetes. If hens have been fed grains, those lectins will end up in the eggs and chicken meat you eat, thus avoid. Unfortunately, many "free-range" eggs come from mostly grain fed hens. About 50 to 80 percent of your diet should be raw or steamed food.

Some authors recommend eating dark chocolate for the health benefits of cocoa powder. It should be sugar-free (like Keto Barks from ChocZero, https://www.choczero.com/). A word of caution: If you have prediabetes or type 2 diabetes, the heated fats in chocolate could worsen your insulin resistance. You could still benefit from cocoa powder if used to make fat bombs (e.g., cocoa powder and coconut oil (or coconut butter or cream), sweetened with monk fruit, allulose, stevia, inulin or a combination thereof; may add a small amount of peppermint and/or cinnamon). You may also use cocoa butter but melt it at a low temperature (110 degrees Fahrenheit).

Reduce phytic acid present in nuts and seeds by soaking, sprouting, or fermenting them. If you dry the nuts, do it at the lower temperature possible to avoid damaging their fats.

At least two-thirds of plant foods should be above-the-ground produce. Minimize underground produce if you have prediabetes or type 2 diabetes until your insulin sensitivity has normalized.

1.9. EAT A LECTIN-FREE DIET OR AT LEAST MINIMIZE LECTINS.

AVOID ALL lectins if you have an autoimmune disease (e.g., multiple sclerosis, rheumatoid arthritis, fibromyalgia, etc.). Some lectins can be destroyed by pressure cooking (e.g., legumes, nightshade vegetables) but others cannot (e.g., grains).

beans, lentils, peas, wheat, soybeans

1.10. OMEGA 6 TO OMEGA 3 RATIO IDEALLY SHOULD BE 1:1.

This is VERY IMPORTANT because to function well, healthy cells need a normal ratio of omega 6:3 fatty acids. The omega 6 to omega 3 fatty acids ratio should not be greater than 3:1. AVOID processed or heated omega 3 oils, as they are very heat sensitive and become harmful once oxidized by heat. Avoid most fish oil capsules. Instead buy fish oil or cod liver oil from a reputable known origin. Shrimp may be boiled in very salty water, then add mayonnaise made with avocado oil. Salmon may be "cured" instead of cooked to avoid damaging the omega 3 fatty acids. It takes nine months for all body cells to regenerate their cell membranes. A high omega 6:3 ratio has been found to correlate with heart disease and type 2 diabetes.

1.11. PROTEIN INTAKE.

Only eat whatever is the amount of protein you need, which is variable based on age and other factors. In general, some protein should be from animal origin to avoid essential amino acids deficiencies. It would take quite a bit of knowledge to eat all essential amino acids on a vegan diet. The official protein RDA (recommended dietary allowance) is 0.8 g/kg/day but this amount varies depending on several circumstances. Nevertheless, it is easier to reverse type 2 diabetes on a pure plant-based diet. Other options are: (a) drinking fat-free bone broth supplemented with essential amino acids; and/or (b) take some whey protein supplements. Protein intake without fat does not increase or decrease the risk of type 2 diabetes.

1.12. DAIRY PRODUCTS.

Dairy products are controversial at best. Goat milk, goat cheese, and sugar-free goat yogurt might be acceptable in small amounts if you are not trying to lose weight. Avoid dairy products if you have prediabetes or type 2 diabetes because insulin sensitivity is worsened by saturated animal fats.

1.13. COOK AT LOW TEMPERATURES.

This is VERY IMPORTANT. It is better not to heat any oils, although coconut oil might be an exception but why take any chances? Why would you buy expensive healthy oils, like extra virgin olive oil, just to make it toxic during cooking? Ideally, cook without any oils and add the oils later. Steaming vegetables is safe. Animal products can be cooked using a Sous Vide water bath or in a crock pot, thus at a significant lower temperature than traditional cooking methods. Although saturated animal fats are more heat stable, when cooked at higher temperatures they increase the risk of type 2 diabetes and hypertension. When oil reaches its smoke point, it has become completely toxic and should be discarded because it has many carcinogens (cancer causing substance). Nevertheless, be careful because oils can become unhealthy way before reaching their smoking point and the exact temperature is not known.

1.14. SUPPORT YOUR GUT MICROBIOME AND PREVENT OR REVERSE A "LEAKY GUT."

This is VERY IMPORTANT. An unhealthy gut microbiome (bacteria, viruses, and fungi in the gut) can cause many diseases. Unhealthy food will cause a "leaky gut" or intestinal permeability (wholes in the lining of the intestines) leading to all types of autoimmune conditions and multiple other medical problems like obesity, inflammatory bowel disease, metabolic syndrome, insulin resistance/diabetes, and mental and behavioral problems. Avoid all emulsifiers, which are found in many processed foods, because they are not good for the bowel mucosa (lining). Examples of emulsifiers are lecithin (often from soy), polysorbate 60 and 80 (made out of petroleum, avoid at any cost), carrageenan, carboxymethylcellulose, xanthan gum, mono- and diglycerides of fatty acids, stearoyl lactylates, sucrose esters, and polyglycerol polyricinoleate. From a practical point of view, the only way to avoid emulsifiers is by not eating processed foods.

Avoid broad spectrum antibiotics if possible. AVOID GLYPHOSATE because it is an antibiotic that kills the good gut bacteria/microbes. Glyphosate is the main ingredient of the herbicide Round Up® and most GMO foods come with it. Glyphosate is also used to spray some non-GMO crops before harvesting them. You can avoid glyphosate by eating organic products.

Your body needs health bacteria supplements/foods (probiotics) and fiber for the bacteria to multiply in the guts (prebiotics). Probiotics in oral form or enemas are useful.

1.15. HYDRATION.

Stay well hydrated by drinking filtered water or tea. Do not drink water with fluoride or chlorine. Coffee is acceptable but drink it in moderation. Do not drink any fruit juices, soda, soft drinks, sports drinks, or energy drinks. Do not drink from any plastic bottles, certainly if they are not BPA free. Always use stainless steel or glass bottles instead.

1.16. SWEETENERS.

Avoid ALL artificial sweeteners (aspartame/Nutrasweet, sucralose/Splenda, and saccharine). Minimize or avoid alcoholic sugars. Some sweeteners are safe, like allulose, monk fruit, inulin, and stevia. Buy the organic options.

1.17. BLOOD CHOLESTEROL AND CHOLESTEROL INTAKE.

Cholesterol in food neither increases the "bad" cholesterol in the blood (the small dense LDL particles) nor causes heart attacks. Saturated animal fats do increase total cholesterol and LDL some but mostly the good LDL (A particles, the larger fluffy ones) and HDL (also called "good" cholesterol). Total cholesterol and LDL, often used to prescribe statin medications, are not reliable predictors of heart disease. Use other tests instead, like high sensitive CRP (C-reactive protein), the ratio triglyceride/HDL, particulate LDL, fibrinogen, homocysteine, or a cardiac scan if indicated. Also check a vitamin D level since low levels correlate with higher risk of heart disease. Heart attacks and other degenerative diseases are caused by chronic inflammation not cholesterol intake. Heart disease is mostly caused by a combination of chronic inflammation with other contributing factors like vitamin K2 deficiency (do not confuse with vitamin K1) and a magnesium deficiency at the cellular level.

1.18. ALCOHOL.

Avoid or minimize with the possible exception of red wine. Do not start drinking if you are not a drinker because some people have a genetic predisposition to become alcoholics.

1.19. SALT INTAKE.

Excessive intake of salt (sodium chloride) can cause high blood pressure. The solution is simple. Avoid too much salt by not eating any processed foods, which are the biggest single source of unhealthy salt intake (about 75 percent). Both sodium and chloride are essential, thus necessary for normal life. A truly "salt sensitive" person will need to eat less salt to control his or her blood pressure. Most people eating mostly a whole food plant diet can use salt as needed. Avoid the usual "table salt" because it has been bleached, lacks other minerals, and comes with anticaking agents. Instead, buy Mediterranean, Celtic Sea, Himalayan, or Redmond salts. All these salts have minute amounts of other minerals (trace minerals) which the body needs to maintain healthy bones. If your blood pressure is high, the first thing to do is to take magnesium (400 mg to 1000 mg/day) and potassium supplements for a few weeks. Often blood pressure will normalize. You may need to decrease or stop your current blood pressure medication, so monitor your blood pressure carefully. People are often mislabeled as "salt sensitive" because they have an intracellular deficiency of magnesium and/or potassium. A hair tissue mineral analysis will clarify this issue.

Sodium bicarbonate (baking soda) does not have chloride and does NOT increase blood pressure.

1.20. BONE BROTH.

Bone broth is very healthy. Chicken bone broth is good for joint cartilage because it has type 2 collagen. Beef bone broth has types 1 and 3 collagen and it benefits the skin.

1.21. KETOGENIC VS NON-KETOGENIC DIET.

An eco ketogenic diet is healthy but not mandatory. A ketogenic diet should be low in net carbohydrates (50 grams or less) but normal amount of protein. Net carbohydrates are total carbohydrates minus grams of fiber. It has some indications like children with epilepsy, cancer patients, management of diabetes, and for weight loss. A ketogenic diet should NOT be high in animal protein as many people think. A high animal protein ketogenic diet is harmful in the long run even though might be helpful to lose weight in the short term. For a ketogenic diet to be healthy, it must be eco ketogenic diet (plant-based). Fat bombs can be used to increase the percentage of fat intake.

1.22. TYPE 2 DIABETES MELLITUS.

MUST AVOID all (a) bad fats and oils and (b) heated fats and oils.

Type 2 diabetes is usually not due a lack of insulin (like type 1 diabetes) but due to insulin resistance. Plenty of insulin available (except in the late stages of the disease) but the insulin receptor does not work well, thus glucose accumulates in the blood because it does not enter muscle cells and other cells.

This disease is CAUSED BY FAT not sugar (few exceptions might exist). Saturated animal fats are the main culprit or at least are the better studied with more supporting evidence. Other contributing fats are trans fats (hydrogenated oils), man-made fats (e.g., interesterified fats), and processed vegetable oils. Interesterified fats were the worse for glucose control in one study (highest risk of developing diabetes).

All heated fats or oils, even the healthy ones, can cause or worsen type 2 diabetes because they increase insulin resistance. This is why in some studies type 2 diabetic patients were able to control their blood sugars better on a high carbohydrate but low fat diet.

1.23. OBESITY

EATING FAT DOES NOT MAKE YOU FAT, refined carbohydrates do. Rule out endocrine and toxic conditions. Then start a plant-based ketogenic diet. Initially avoid all animal products and alcohol. You should have a home glucometer and find out how specific meals are affecting your 2-hour and 3-hour post meal blood sugar (glucose). Fasting and intermittent fasting help weight loss.

2. FASTING. CALORIE RESTRICTED DIET VS. FASTING.

VERY IMPORTANT. Periodic fasting is one of the MOST EFFECTIVE WAYS TO STAY HEALTHY. It does not take any time or sophisticated knowledge and it is free. It has very few contraindications, like malnourishment, pregnancy, and breastfeeding. It has not been studied for children in the USA but low calorie diets since birth have been found safe in many animal studies. Some patients, like persons with diabetes or hypertension, should be medically monitored. Fasting has been successfully used in conjunction with chemotherapy.

A 5-day fast rejuvenates the body by increasing circulating stem cells. It also stimulates autophagia, the process by which cells recycle old organelles. A fast mimicking diet, as proposed by Dr. Valter Longo, is equivalent to the old fashioned fast—water fast or less than 400 calories/day—although weight loss might be less. Dr. Longo has predicted chronic degenerative conditions could be decreased in half if 5-day fasting was used periodically. Fasting also allows old and unhealthy cells to die (apoptosis) before becoming cancerous.

Calorie restriction has been shown to always improve health and prolong life expectancy in many animal studies. It was the best option a few decades ago. But it has some side effects and, for most people, it has become obsolete because repeated intermittent fasting offers superior results and benefits, and it is easier to implement. From a practical point of view, most people are not able follow a chronic calorie restricted diet.

3. EXERCISE.

Exercise and remaining physically active is A MUST. The best exercise is HIIT (high intensity interval training), it has more health benefits and is less time consuming than pure aerobic exercise. HIIT combines aerobic with anaerobic exercise. During and after losing weight, exercise is needed to maintain a normal metabolic rate which invariably drops with weight loss. It would be almost impossible to keep the weight off if the metabolic rate decreased significantly, which is what happens with traditional caloric restriction weight loss (the so-called "portion control"). HIIT also increases the secretion of growth hormone.

Resistance training (e.g., weight lifting and similar exercises) is also very good. It is ideal to maintain or increase muscle mass. Thus, it is very helpful for older people who should try to at least maintain their muscle strength. Unfortunately, aerobic exercise will not prevent the decline of muscle mass.

Some authors feel exercise while fasting provides additional health benefits.

4.   CONTROL CHRONIC STRESS

In the long term, chronic stress is extremely harmful. It will release a larger amount of cortisol and will deplete intracellular magnesium. High levels of cortisol (a stress hormone) negatively impact the whole body, including the immune system, increasing the risk of heart attacks, hypertension, cancers, etc. Chronic stress depletes magnesium, a mineral essential in energy production. A chronic magnesium deficiency increases the risk of developing many health problems, like heart attacks, high blood pressure, muscle cramps, restless leg syndrome, insomnia, osteoporosis, chronic fatigue, and fibromyalgia.

Meditation is the best way to control chronic stress. Other options include yoga, deep breathing, and Reiki. Wim Hof has a protocol that includes deep breathing exercises and cold showers, which also increases brown fat.

5.   AVOID TOXINS AND DETOXIFY

5.1. AVOID ENVIRONMENTAL TOXINS.

Unfortunately, this is easier said than done, but do your best. Do not expose yourself to any pesticides.

5.2. COOKING HARDWARD AND FOOD STORAGE.

Avoid aluminum, teflon/non-stick, and copper. Use stainless steel, ceramic or ceramic coated.

For food storage, use glass.

5.3. DEODORANTS

Avoid antiperspirant in general and any deodorant with aluminum. For a review of healthy personal hygiene products you may visit www.ewg.org

5.4. ORAL HYGIENE

Use a good prebiotic fluoride-free toothpaste, like Revitin, and floss frequently to avoid gingivitis, which increases heart disease.

5.5. SKIN PRODUCTS.

Always use organic skin products. Do not apply a cosmetic product to your skin if you are not willing to eat those ingredients.
Use glycerin based soaps and organic detergents.

5.6. DETOXIFY REGULARLY.

The world is very polluted and it is not possible for people to remain toxicant free regardless how much they try. Thus, you must detoxify your body from man-made pollutants on a chronic basis. Several protocols are available as described later.

6. CANCER PREVENTION AND CANCER RECURRENCE PREVENTION.

VERY IMPORTANT. Most cancers are preventable (like heart disease is) by understanding epigenetics. Alkalize your body, avoid hormonal disrupters, minimize stimulating the mTOR genetic pathway by avoiding excess protein in general, and more specifically animal protein. Avoid toxins like smoking cigarettes, food cooked at high temperatures, pesticides, etc. Several supplements are available to improve your immune system and prevent cancers in general. The inexpensive SODIUM BICARBONATE (baking soda) is probably the most effective cancer prevention intervention in addition to avoiding carcinogens (like smoking, excess sun exposure, etc.) and eating a healthy diet.

7. OTHER RECOMMENDATIONS

7.1. MICROWAVE OVENS.

Avoid cooking meals in microwave ovens because the food will lose nutritional value. It seems reasonable to use microwave ovens occasionally to reheat meals. This will not produce any toxic products like it happens when food is overheated on the stove or in a traditional oven.

7.2. GROUNDING (EARTHING).

Best grounding is walking barefoot on the beach with the sun shining on your skin. At home, use a copper rod inserted in the ground by your house.

7.3. CIRCADIAN RHYTHM.

Sleep 8 hours a day, always going to bed at about the same time. All body cells have a circadian rhythm. Avoid blue light at night and realize it might cause retinal damage (thus increasing the risk of macular degeneration and blindness).

7.4. LED LIGHTS.

LED are very disruptive. They interfere with normal circadian rhythms if used at night because of their blue light spectrum.

In addition, some scientific evidence indicates LED lights may permanently harm the retina (French government, Madrid Complutense study, etc.).

7.5. DONATE BLOOD IF ABLE.

Donate blood at least once a year. It decreases the risk of heart disease among other health benefits.

7.6. AMALGAMS WITH MERCURY.

This is a very controversial issue. I would leave the amalgams (dental fillings) alone (do not remove them) as long as you do not have any mercury poisoning symptoms and your hair tissue mineral analysis does not show any toxic levels. Removal of amalgams that have mercury carries a significant risk of mercury poisoning. If you decide to replace your silver amalgam fillings, go to a dentist who has the appropriate suctioning equipment and expertise in this procedure.

7.7. VACCINES IN GENERAL.

Do your research since this has become a political issue with big corporate financial interests at stake. Suffice it to say that too much of any good thing can end up having serious side effects.

7.8. INLUENZA VACCINE.

Carefully balance the risks against the benefits of the flu shot (influenza vaccine).

7.9. AUTISM.

Stay away from the combination of aluminum-glyphosate because it is the main cause of autism. This combination also contributes to dementia. Thus, do not eat any GMO food. Do not take any shots or vaccines that have aluminum (or mercury) in them. Do not expose your body to any aluminum

7.10. SUNLIGHT AND EXPOSURE.

Sunlight has many health benefits, some probably still unknown. Like with anything else, moderation is the key. Excessive sunlight is the main cause of skin cancers, as well as wrinkles and premature skin aging. Exposure of a large percentage of the body to midday sunlight for 15 to 20 minutes per day is enough. This will produce several thousand units of vitamin D, which is never toxic when obtained this natural way. Some sunlight is good for retinal health.

7.11. BROWN FAT.

Brown fat is seen in infants but then the amount decreases with age. Increasing the amount of the body's brown fat amount is healthy. Brown fat is metabolically very active. In other words, it uses energy. Thus, it keeps you warm and also helps losing weight. The most effective way to increase brown fat is exposure to cold temperatures. For example, take a 2- to 4-minute cold shower daily. Do your best if you are willing to try, and good luck trying to stick to this routine.

8. RECOMMENDATIONS FOR AUTOIMMUNE DISEASES

Although not "curable", many autoimmune diseases can be controlled with simple common sense measures. The underlying genetic predisposition cannot be cured but the triggering mechanisms can be discontinued.

9. PAIN KILLERS.

Avoid NASAIDS, like ibuprofen and naproxen. Also avoid acetaminophen if you can. You may use Boswellia instead. NSAIDS have many side effects and worsen the leaky gut problem. They also negatively affect cartilage, thus worsening osteoarthritis. Another safe pain killer option is white willow bark. As an anti-inflammatory medication, use turmeric.

10. SUPPLEMENTS (SOME ARE VERY IMPORTANT)

10.1. SUPPLEMENTS IN GENERAL

10.1.1. VITAMIN C

10.1.2. MAGNESIUM

10.1.3. VITAMIN D3

10.1.4. VITAMIN K2

10.1.5. MULTIVITAMINS/MINERALS

10.1.6. OMEGA 3 FATTY ACIDS

10.1.7. CALCIUM

10.1.8. SUPPLEMENTS TO IMPROVE CELL ENERGY PRODUCTION

10.2. SUPPLEMENTS FOR SPECIFIC CONDITIONS

10.2.1. HEART HEALTH

10.2.2. ARTERIOSCLEROSIS/ATHEROSCLEROSIS

10.2.3. FOR VEGANS

10.2.4. HIGH BLOOD PRESSURE (HYPERTENSION)

10.2.5. WEIGHT LOSS

10.2.6. CATARACTS

10.2.7. OSTEOPOROSIS

10.2.8. ERECTILE DYSFUNCTION

10.2.9. FIBROMYALGIA

10.2.10. ATRIAL FIBRILLATION

11. STUDIES

11.1. LABORATORY STUDIES (SERUM/BLOOD)

High sensitive CRP, fasting glucose, 2-hour post meal glucose, Hgb A1c, lipid panel, fasting insulin level, vitamin D level, and ferritin. High sensitive CRP (C-reactive protein) predicts heart disease better then cholesterol. It is also known as cardiac CRP. High triglycerides increase the risk of heart disease and are usually due to overconsumption of carbohydrates as well as trans fats (hydrogenated or partially hydrogenated oils).

Other studies may be ordered based on personal factors (e.g., rule out hypothyroidism, insulin resistance, heavy metal toxicity, etc.)

11.2. CARDIAC SCAN (CORONARY ARTERY CALCIUM SCORE).

11.3. HAIR ANALYSIS (HTMA – HAIR TISSUE MINERAL ANALYSIS)

11.4. BONE DENSITY SCAN

12. FUNCTIONAL MEDICINE

13. DOCUMENTARIES

14. OTHER REFERENCES

14.1. CANCER AND SODIUM BICARBONATE (BAKING SODA)

14.2. EARTHING OR GROUNDING

14.3. BLOOD DONATION

15. ALTERNATIVE THERAPIES FOR CANCER TREATMENT AND OTHER DISEASES

15.1. GCMAF

15.2. CHLORINE DIOXIDE THERAPY

15.3. HULDA REGEHR CLARK, PH.D, TREATMENT PROTOCOL FOR CANCER

15.4. KETOGENIC DIET WITH GLUTAMINE INHIBITORS

15.5. FENBENDAZOLE

15.6. DCA THERAPY

15.7. VITAMIN B17

15.8. SODIUM BICARBONATE

15.9. FIVE-DAY FAST

15.10. ELECTROMAGNETIC FREQUENCY THERAPY

DETAILED EXPLANATION

1. RECOMMENDATIONS FOR FOOD AND COOKING

1.1. AVOID PROCESSED FOODS.

Again, this is the MOST IMPORTANT change you can make. Exceptions include single food products (e.g., extra virgin olive oil, organic coconut oil, olives, etc.) that come in a healthy container (e.g., glass, BPA-free can, etc.). If you buy any processed foods, carefully read the ingredient list to make sure no harmful products are included like natural flavors, MSG, emulsifiers, high fructose corn syrup, any type of sugar (about 50 different names are being used), any artificial sweetener, etc. Emulsifiers harm the lining of the bowel (bowel mucosa) increasing the risk of developing a "leaky gut." You will need to do extensive research to figure out what ingredients are harmful.

The food industry goal is maximizing profits NOT improving your health. Their logo for some time was or has been "convenience" but how inconvenient will it be when you become ill and start suffering from chronic medical conditions?

Most processed foods come with very unhealthy processed vegetable oils, which increase heart disease and diabetes. In addition, they often have many unhealthy preservatives or chemicals. About 80 percent have MSG (mono sodium glutamate) in some form or another (more than 50 different names are used) which is harmful and increases appetite (you may Google "MSG induced rat obesity") and negatively affects the brain. Many other unhealthy ingredients like preservatives, sugar, artificial sweeteners, etc., are found in processed food. Sugar increases their addictive qualities and the food industry is well aware of this fact. The nutritional value of processed foods is significantly decreased.

Avoid any products with added fructose, high fructose corn syrup, sugar or sucrose—beware, there are 56 names for sugar. If you do not know what the ingredient is or how to pronounce it, avoid it.

Processed foods promote many chronic conditions, like heart disease, type 2 diabetes, hypertension, etc. Nitrates and nitrates, frequently found in cured meats and deli in general, have been found to increase the risk of colorectal cancer.

Thus, COOK YOUR OWN MEALS with organic whole fresh foods instead of eating out or eating processed food at home. Southern European countries often used a quick homemade salad dressing by combining extra virgin olive oil with some vinegar and salt.

Avoid ALL "reduced fat" or "fat free" versions of a normal product (e.g., skim or low fat milk). People choosing low fat products end up eating too many carbohydrates. Many of those carbohydrates are refined (like bread, pasta, pizza, etc.) and, thus, much worse than healthy fats.
Pertinent sources/books:

- *Timbebome. A Genocide of DEADLY Processed Foods!* by Joe Horn.
- *What's Making Our Children SICK? How Industrial Food Is Causing an Epidemic of Chronic Illness, and What Parents (and Doctors) Can Do About It* by Michelle Perro, MD and Vincanne Adams, PhD.
- *Fat for Fuel* by Dr. Joseph Mercola.
- *The Plant Paradox* by Dr. Steven R. Gundry.
- *FAT Chance. Beating the Odds Against SUGAR, PROCESSED FOOD, OBESITY, and DISEASE* by Robert H. Lustig, MD.
- *Salt Sugar Fat: How the Food Giants Hooked Us* by Michael Moss.

1.2. EAT GOOD FATS BUT AVOILD ALL BAD FATS.

This is CRITICAL to remain healthy. You should avoid all bad fats, NO EXCEPTIONS. Bad fats are quite pro-inflammatory and worse to your health than tobacco. If you do not smoke because is very harmful, there is no reason why you should not ban all bad fats from your diet. Believe or not, bad fats are worse than sugar/s because no amount is safe. Oil is a fat in liquid form at room temperature.

We can divide fats into three types: (a) bad fats; (b) healthy fats; and (c) healthy fats that have turned toxic for various reasons like subjected to increased temperatures, oxidized, or if they become rancid. In the real world, it is more complicated because healthy fats can negatively affect or even cause some conditions, like type 2 diabetes.

A good review of good versus bad fats can be found in the classic book *Fats that Heal, Fats that Kill* by Udo Erasmus.

Bad fats include all man-made trans fats (also called hydrogenated or partially hydrogenated oils), all man-made artificial fats (e.g., Crisco, margarines, interesterified fats), and all processed vegetable oils (canola, corn, cottonseed, sunflower, soy, safflower). Peanut oil is somewhat less harmful but I would avoid it because it has lectins. All man-made fats, like trans fats, are not well metabolized in the body and cause heart disease, heart attacks, strokes, and type 2 diabetes. The above vegetable oils are highly processed, heated, treated with chemicals, and have a large percentage of the pro-inflammatory omega 6 fatty acids. Avoid them all.

The FDA allows labeling zero trans fats when the amount contained per serving is less than 0.5 grams. Often people eat more than one serving. With time, trans fat consumption will add up if you eat process foods. No amount of trans fats is safe. This is another good reason for avoiding processed foods all together.

In general, omega 6 fatty acids are pro-inflammatory with the exception of GLA (gamma-linolenic acid) which does not increase inflammation and is healthy. Although omega 6 is an essential fat, in excess it becomes quite harmful. The typical American diet has a very high and unhealthy omega 6:3 ratio.

Healthy fats or oils include omega 3 fatty acids, cold-pressed avocado oil, extra virgin olive oil, organic coconut oil, macadamia oil, sesame seed oil, flax seed oil, hemp oil, almond oil, and walnut oil. But be careful because all refined oils, even of those oils mentioned, are unhealthy and should be avoided.

Raw nuts and seeds are very healthy. They have healthy oils and vitamins, as well minerals. But roasted nuts and seeds are unhealthy due to heat changes suffered by fat during roasting.

Saturated animal fats (like butter or lard) are safe in general but should not be abused because they are somewhat pro-inflammatory. Animal fats do not cause coronary heart disease (heart disease or heart attacks), as it has been well proven by a large body of scientific evidence. Thus, there is no longer an official maximum recommended daily allowance for cholesterol intake. Nevertheless, saturated animal fats are only healthy from animals pasture-raised or free-range which were not given ANY grain feedings. It is even worse if the animals were fed GMO grains which come with pesticides, like glyphosate. Some products advertise grass-fed but the animals have been fed grains towards the end (to increase the animal weight quickly). Thus, it should be an animal not given any grains. Also, free-range does not exclude possible grain feedings, thus research the product you are buying. Grain-fed animals have a much higher percentage of pro-inflammatory omega 6 fatty acids while grass-fed animals have a higher percentage of anti-inflammatory omega 3 fatty acids. Although saturated animal fats do not increase the risk of heart disease, they do not decrease the risk like other fats/oils do (e.g., olive oil, healthy nuts, etc.) Saturated animal fats, as well as animal protein, should not be abused. In addition, saturated animal fats increase the risk of type 2 diabetes, thus prediabetics and diabetics should not eat them. Whether an exception can be made for unheated saturated animal fats is something we do not have a final answer yet.

Coconut oil is mostly a saturated fat. I have not found any studies linking coconut oil to insulin resistance or type 2 diabetes. Limited data from animal and human studies do indicate coconut oil is safe, and it may even decrease the risk of type 2 diabetes.

Saturated animal fats are much more resistant to heating than other oils and this also applies to coconut oil. This is why some experts recommend coconut oil for cooking. A word of caution: any oil or fat will become unhealthy if heated enough.

1.3. AVOID, OR AT LEAST MINIMIZE, EATING OUT AT RESTAURANTS.

Some experts have estimated about 40-45 percent of total food cost in the USA is spent eating out. Restaurants focus on portions and good tasting meals, not on health.

Most restaurant cook with unhealthy oils and/or at high temperatures. Many restaurants —if not most—reuse cooking vegetable oils time after time, which is a very harmful practice because every time oil is heated it becomes more unhealthy. Every time oil is heated enough, it becomes more oxidized thus increasing the amount of unhealthy (small particle) LDL in the blood. You should not routinely eat at restaurants in general and much less at fast food restaurants. If you do, only do it as an exception for special occasions and go to a restaurant that offers healthy choices. You do not have much or any control over what happens in the restaurant kitchen.

In short, cook your own meals at home. All the money you will save can be used to purchase healthy organic foods.

1.4. DO NOT EAT ANY SUGAR OR REFINED CARBOHYDRATES.

VERY IMPORTANT. Refined carbohydrates do not exist in nature and are quite harmful to your health. They greatly increase the risk of heart attacks which is the leading cause of early deaths. Sugar and refined carbohydrates are pro-inflammatory. Sugar is a main contributor to heart attacks and arterial diseases, like strokes. It decreases your body's pH, as excess animal protein will also do. Chronic inflammation is the root of all chronic conditions, including heart attacks and cancer. By lowering the body's pH, cancer cells and viruses will grow more easily. The body will try to buffer the pH by "robbing" precious minerals from the bones, thus leading to osteoporosis. Sugar and refined carbohydrates cause obesity. Modern western diets high in sugar and refined carbohydrates are clearly responsible for our current obesity epidemic and are contributor to chronic degenerative diseases.

In addition, this type of western diet has also been linked to type 2 diabetes (even though carbohydrates are not the actual or main cause).

Moreover, sugar and refined carbohydrates are nutrient depleted. It is difficult getting all necessary nutrients while eating a healthy diet. It would be almost impossible when eating nutrient depleted foods. The food industry statement "a calorie is a calorie", when talking about weight control and calorie intake, is totally incorrect (I am being polite by avoiding the word "lie") from a metabolic point of view because the way different foods are metabolized and used by the body.

So, why is it so difficult to stop eating sugar? Because sugar creates a strong addiction by stimulating the same brain center that is stimulated by cocaine. In an experimental study, rats given sugar and cocaine chose sugar. Carbohydrates in general will allow some specific gut bacteria to flourish. These bacteria will communicate with the brain, via the vagus nerve/s or via intravenous chemicals, and will request more carbohydrates. Those cravings will completely subside once the culprit bacteria have been starved on a low carbohydrate, sugar-free diet.

All refined carbohydrates should be avoided, including pasta, bread, pastries, bagels, cookies, crackers, pizza, all flours, etc. Rice, although not as harmful, should be avoided or at least minimized because it also has lectins. Wild rice is considered better by some experts but others disagree because of its lectin content. Thus, if you eat wild rice do so in moderation.

Avoid any products with added fructose, high fructose corn syrup, sugar or sucrose—beware. There are 56 names for sugar. If you do not know what the ingredient is or how to pronounce it, avoid it.

In general, minimize food products that decrease the body's pH. A good source of information is the book *Alkalize or Die* from Dr. Theodore A. Baroody.

1.5. MINIMIZE FRUCTOSE.

Fructose (sugar is half fructose) is a metabolic poison which in larger amounts is quite harmful to the human body. As mentioned, it causes fatty liver disease (and cirrhosis), hepatic (liver) insulin resistance (which increases the risk of diabetes), and increases obesity risk and uric acid (which can cause gout) among other conditions. It also increases triglycerides, which increase heart disease (heart attacks).

Fructose is found in fruits and the food industry loves it because it is cheaper and sweeter than sugar. High fructose corn syrup is usually made from GMO corn, thus it is even worse because in addition to the fructose it comes with significant amounts of pesticides, like glyphosate. Our bodies are not design to handle or metabolize large amounts of fructose. The ongoing epidemic of fatty liver disease is mostly due to the increased consumption of fructose.

Fruits are meant to be eaten when they are in season. Fructose in fruits also comes with fiber which decreases its negative effects. In large amounts, as frequently as people eat or drink, fruits become unhealthy. Dr. Robert H. Lustig has written a nice review of fructose—and processed food—in his book *FAT Chance. Beating the Odds Against Sugar, Processed Food, Obesity, and Disease.* You can also watch on YouTube his video *Sugar: The Bitter Truth.* https://www.youtube.com/watch?v=dBnniua6-oM

Added sugar or fructose become toxic very quickly and some researchers think it increases the risk of type 2 diabetes mellitus and other degenerative diseases. See *Is a Calorie a Calorie? Processed Food, Experiment Gone Wrong* on YouTube. Dr. Lustig—a pediatric endocrinologists—recommends keeping daily added sugar to no more than 6 teaspoons for women and 9 teaspoons for men: *What Is Metabolic Syndrome, and Why Are Children Getting It* https://www.youtube.com/watch?v=UEA6ow1icDc).

All fruit juices should be avoided because they have too much sugar.

Do not buy any foods with added sugar or fructose. It is acceptable to eat one or two pieces of fruit per day. Ideally, fruit should be eaten from a local producer only when it is in season. One apple a day is acceptable, ideally a granny apple because it has less fructose. Berries in general, and blueberries specifically, are very healthy.

Pomegranate juice (or powder) has been shown to improve carotid stenosis (narrowing of the large artery in the neck). Avoid, or at least minimize, dried fruits with high fructose content, like raisins.

The best recommendation is not to "eat fruits and vegetables" but to eat many vegetables (only a small percentage of root vegetables) and some fruits.

1.6. DO NOT EAT ANY GLUTEN AND AVOID ALL GRAINS.

Gluten is found not just in wheat but also in rye, barley, most beers, etc.

Gluten is a neurotoxin (damages nerves), and it should be COMPLETELY AVOIDED. Besides being a contributor to dementia, gluten will cause ataxia (unstable gate, falls) because it damages the cerebellum. It takes about 5 decades for the neurotoxic effect to start showing up. Once nerve damage has occurred, though, it is irreversible.

Gluten stimulates appetite and increases daily calorie intake by several hundred calories—about 400 calories/day—because increases appetite by stimulating the brain. This fact has been known for many decades.

✳ Gluten causes a leaky gut, which increases chronic inflammation and many autoimmune conditions.

Gluten has "morphine like" properties, thus it will take some effort to get over the cravings.

Possible exception for ancient wheat, like Einkorn. The DNA of ancient gluten is quite different and smaller compared to modern wheat. Einkorn only has 14 chromosomes compared to 42 for modern wheat. At least one animal study showed modern wheat harms the gut lining causing leaky gut (intestinal permeability), which will lead to many health problems including autoimmune diseases, heart attacks, etc. But in the same study ancient wheat did not damage the gut lining. We do not have any long term data to decide whether or not ancient gluten is neurotoxic (thus contributing to unstable gate and dementia). Furthermore, it has lectins. Thus, eat in moderation if at all.

Good information about gluten can be found in *Grain Brain* by Dr. David Perlmutter—neurologist—and *Wheat Belly* by Dr. William Davis—cardiologist.

All grains have unhealthy lectins (a protein plans use to defend themselves from predators), even the so called "healthy" grains like quinoa. Lectins in grains cannot be destroyed by pressure cooking. Anybody with an autoimmune disease should avoid them.

1.7. CONSUME ORGANIC FOODS.

It seems many consumers are effectively "brainwashed" into spending as little as possible on food. A person buying an expensive car will probably not even consider filling up the gas tank with an ultra cheap and poor quality gasoline or fuel. Why would intelligent people do so when "filling up" (feeding) their own bodies, which they need to enjoy a good life? It is acceptable in society to buy an expensive car or to eat out frequently. But many people frown when told to buy healthy organic food because is more expensive.

Non-organic food per definition comes with many more pesticides, some of them quite unhealthy. The most notorious one, due to its very extensive use, is glyphosate (the main herbicide in Round Up®). It has been linked to many diseases or conditions, including autism, auto-immune diseases, several cancers, dementia, etc. Non-organic crops tend to be mono-crops and use petroleum derived fertilizers which harm the quality of the soil. In fact, the overuse of those petroleum based fertilizers depletes the soil from nutrients because it harms normal soil bacteria. Processed foods further decrease the remaining nutritional value. The harmful side effects of processed foods are compounded because unhealthy preservatives are added.

Organic foods are grown in a sustainable way and are more resistant to droughts and bad weather. After decades, in at least two farms, the long-term yield in organic farms is not any smaller then non-organic standard commercial farming. If the food product is organic, it cannot have been sprayed with glyphosate and must be BPA-free. Organic farming allows multiple soil bacteria to proliferate. Bacteria byproducts feed the plants, making them more nutritious for human consumption.

Long-term, organic food is not more expensive. In fact, it will save you money and quite a bit of physical and emotional suffering in the long run. In short, AVOID ALL GM foods.

Eat an organic diet (called biologic or ecologic in other countries), mostly plant-based, with large amounts of fresh vegetables of different colors (including a large amount of green leafy vegetables) and some fruits. The best way to do so is by blending the vegetables. Juicing is not ideal since the fiber is lost, with few exceptions like celery juice treatments. Add cold water or cold iced green tea and drink it shortly after blending. It tastes better if ice is blended in, also if one apple is added. Some fruits maybe used frozen (e.g., grapes). Some nutritionists discourage adding fruits to vegetables, maybe with the exception of apples. Fruits are healthy but initially when reversing chronic conditions, like type 2 diabetes, should be limited to one or two per day (berries may be eaten in addition). Even without prediabetes it is reasonable to avoid excess fruit intake. Ideally, only in season fruits should be eaten. Buy a good quality blender. You may add to the smoothie healthy food products like chlorella, spirulina, cilantro, avocado, nuts, raw sesame seeds, and seaweed. The smoothie base may consist of green vegetables like kale, collard, spinach, and celery. Hemp protein powder can be used to increase the amount of protein (hemp protein has several advantages over whey protein) but do not eat excess protein. Stevia, inulin, or monk fruit can be added for better flavor.

A significant percentage of calories can be from organic raw nuts (unsalted, not toasted) with the exception of cashews, which have lectins. Roasted seeds and nuts are not healthy because the heat negatively affects the quality of the fat. Avoid peanuts, though, as they are legumes not tree nuts and have too many omega 6 fatty acids as well as lectins. Seeds are healthy in general. Sesame seeds have a large amount of calcium and magnesium; both are well absorbed by the body. Do not eat any sprouted seeds from grains that have lectins (e.g., alfalfa). Sprouted broccoli is healthy and can be used for smoothies. Mini greens are usually lectin-free.

You may eat organic legumes if you are not on a ketogenic diet. People eating legumes have been found to have less type 2 diabetes. But you must cook legumes in a pressure cooker to destroy most lectins. An electric pressure cooker is much more convenient than the old cook top pressure cookers.

1.8. EAT MOSTLY A PLANT-BASED DIET.

Eat organic WHOLE FOODS prepared or cooked at home. Most foods should be plant-based and organic.

An IDEAL DIET for persons WITHOUT prediabetes or type 2 diabetes is:

- high on healthy plant-based fats (ideally not heated), no bad fats,
- normal/low protein (only whatever your needs are),
- low or moderate carbohydrate with NO refined or simple carbohydrates. Only carbohydrates found in whole foods. No grains.

A traditional high carbohydrate diet will significantly worsen several health risk factors. See *The Cholesterol Conondrum—and Root Cause Solution* https://www.youtube.com/watch?v=fuj6nxCDBZ0

Although saturated fats from grass-fed or free-range animals do not increase the risk of heart disease, they significantly increase the risk for type 2 diabetes. Again, DO NOT EAT any grain-fed animal products. Excess animal protein increases cancer risk, red meat more than other animal proteins.

FRESH food is much better if you have a choice. Avoid as much as possible canned or frozen products. 50 to 80 percent of your diet should be raw or steamed food.

Some authors recommend eating dark chocolate for the health benefits of cocoa powder. It should be sugar-free (like Keto Barks from ChocZero, https://www.choczero.com/). A word of caution: If you have prediabetes or type 2 diabetes, the heated fats in chocolate could worsen your insulin resistance. You could still benefit from cocoa powder if used to make fat bombs. E.g., cocoa powder and coconut oil (or coconut butter or cream), sweetened with monk fruit, allulose, stevia, inulin or a combination thereof; may add a small amount of peppermint and/or cinnamon. May also use cocoa butter but melt it at very low temperatures (105-110 degrees Fahrenheit) to avoid damaging the fat. Thus, do not place cocoa butter in a pot on the cook top. A food dehydrator or an air fryer will work well.

At least two-thirds of plant foods should be above-the-ground produce. Minimize underground produce if you have prediabetes or type 2 diabetes until your insulin sensitivity has normalized. Then, follow your blood sugars carefully to make sure your blood glucose does not increase much when eating more carbohydrates.

Mushrooms are a fungi, not a vegetable, and are healthy. You may steam mushrooms with salt and then add oil.

Garlic and onions have many health benefits. Use them often in your cooking.

Probiotics. Take daily probiotics supplements if no goat yogurt or other fermented foods are consumed. If goat milk is consumed, it should be from a known source and drink it in moderation but it might be better to avoid it all together. In addition, fermented foods (e.g., sauerkraut) are a must to keep a healthy intestinal flora.

Prebiotics. Prebiotics (e.g., garlic, onions, inulin, etc.) are needed for the probiotics (bacteria) to grow/multiply and work well. Thus, eat daily prebiotics or take them as a nutritional supplement.

Daily fiber intake should be 35 to 50 grams/day (may drink sugar/sweetener-free psyllium, e.g., Konsyl or other brand of organic psyllium).

Animal products. It is difficult, although not impossible, to eat a complete and well balanced diet that includes all essential amino acids when eating vegan. Thus, you may eat healthy fish (usually small fish like sardines, shrimp, etc.) twice a week. This fish will provide you with the needed omega 3 fatty acids. Avoid high temperature cooking. In fact, cured or smoked fish would be the best way to preserve the quality of the omega 3.

Some authors think a small percentage of animal fat and protein from other sources is acceptable. For example, eggs (free range), organic goat cheese, or organic whole goat milk yogurt with live/active cultures (sugar free), grass-fed animals and free range chicken. Animals should not have been fed any grains.

Nevertheless, avoid animal products if you have prediabetes or type 2 diabetes. In this case, though, it is still acceptable to eat egg whites or whey protein to supplement all essential amino acids.

Only 10 to 15 percent of calories should be from animal products. Let me say it again. Although saturated fat from grass-fed or free-range animals does not increase the risk of heart disease, it significantly increases the risk of type 2 diabetes.

Some vegetables can cause hypothyroidism and other problems when eaten raw and should be cooked or steamed even before using them for a smoothie. Vegetables that need to be cooked or steamed include broccoli, Brussels sprouts, cauliflower, broccolini, Bok Choy, radish, Chinese cabbage, spinach, okra, leeks, kale, beet and turnip greens, chard, and collards. Some of these vegetables have goitrogens (a substance that can cause goiter) and/or oxalic acid (can cause kidney stones), which can be neutralized with cooking. If you cook vegetables, do not add oil or fat until they are cooked to prevent fats from deteriorating.

A large percentage of food should be raw or steamed (e.g., vegetables), at least 50 percent but higher for certain conditions like heart disease or type 2 diabetes.

Phytic acid is present in many foods, like seeds and nuts (except for macadamias). Unfortunately, phytic acid will impair the absorption of minerals, like calcium, magnesium, and zinc. Mineral deficiencies will have adverse effects, like osteoporosis. In order to reduce phytic acid in seeds and nuts, you may soak, sprout, or ferment them. The most practical way is to soak seeds and nuts for 4 to 12 hours. Then, you may eat them or dry them in an air fryer or food dehydrator. Drying should be at low temperatures, under 140 degrees Fahrenheit, for up to 12 hours. Once dried, seeds and nuts can be stored as usual. A WORD OF CAUTION: If you have type 2 diabetes, use the lowest drying temperature that will get the job done. Also test a 2-hour and 3-hour post meal blood sugar to make sure the fat in the nuts and seeds is not increasing your insulin resistance. See more details under the diabetes section. Another way to partially counteract phytic acid is by eating a citrus fruit at the same time. For example, add nuts, seeds, and lemon or lime juice to your vegetable smoothie.

You should know whether your diet is deficient in vitamins, minerals, omega 3, magnesium, potassium, etc., and whether you are eating too much protein. A good way to find out is using www.cronometer.com which allows you to enter all your meals and gives you a detailed report.

Still not convinced? Well, think about which terrestrial animals are the biggest strongest. Rhinoceros, elephants, giraffes, bison, cattle, etc. What do they have in common? They do not eat any animal products, only a plant-based diet.

1.9. EAT A LECTIN-FREE DIET OR AT LEAST MINIMIZE LECTINS.

Avoid lectins in general unless they can be destroyed. AVOID ALL lectins if you have an autoimmune disease (e.g., multiple sclerosis, rheumatoid arthritis, fibromyalgia, etc.).

Some lectins can be destroyed by pressure cooking (e.g., legumes, nightshade vegetables) but others cannot (e.g., all grains).

Nightshade vegetables (like tomatoes, eggplants, etc.) can be eaten if pealed and seeds are removed.

Foods with lectins to be avoided in general include:

1   Vegetables: soy and soy products, green beans, sugar snap peas, peas, tofu, edamame, all beans and sprouts, texture vegetable protein, pea protein, alfalfa sprouts. Also tomatoes, bell peppers, zucchini, cucumbers, pumpkins, squash, chili peppers, and eggplant.

2   Nuts and seeds: peanuts (are actual legumes), cashews, chia seeds, pumpkin, sunflower.

3   Oils: peanut, cottonseed, corn, canola, soy, sunflower, safflower, grape seed.

4   Refined carbohydrates: flours, cookies, crackers, sugar, milk and dairy products (unless made from goat milk), pasta (usually made with wheat flower), rice, potatoes, cereals, sugar, agave, maltodextrin, pastry, tortillas, artificial sweeteners (e.g., aspartame, Splenda, saccharine).

5   Fruits: Goji berries, melon.

6   Grains: wheat, rice (wild rice included), buckwheat, popcorn, corn, cornstarch, wheatgrass, barley grass, corn syrup, spelt, kashi, einkorn, barley, rye, quinoa, bulgur, kamut, and oats.

Most cows' milk has the unhealthy casein A-1 protein, which has been linked to many health problems including type 1 diabetes mellitus. Goat milk and some Southern European cows produce casein A-2 protein, which is safe unless you are lactose intolerant. Goat milk does not have casein A-1 protein.

1.10. OMEGA 6 TO OMEGA 3 RATIO IDEALLY SHOULD BE 1:1.

VERY IMPORTANT. Both omega 6 and 3 fatty acids are essential. In other words, humans must include them in their diets to survive. Omega 6 are pro-inflammatory and serve certain functions but are harmful if eaten in excess. Omega 3 are anti-inflammatory. It is critical to keep the omega 6 to omega 3 fatty acid ratio between 1:1 to 2:1, certainly not greater than 3:1. A large ratio, typical in the USA, increases inflammation and chronic conditions (heart attacks, strokes, hypertension, etc.).

Fat from fish is good but it must be wild caught, not farm raised (e.g., non-farmed salmon, sardines—good source for vitamin B12). Minimize large fish, like tuna, since it can have mercury. Good sources of fish omega 3 are cod liver oil, non-farmed salmon, sardines, etc. Organic flax seeds (ground or oil) are a good source of plant-based omega 3. One tablespoon of flax seed oil has 7 to 8 grams of omega 3 fatty acid. Unfortunately, the conversion rate from plant omega 3 (e.g., alpha linoleic acid) to fish omega 3 (e.g., EPA, DPA, and DHA which are the ones the body can use) is rather small and most experts still recommend eating fish omega 3.

Omega 3 fatty acids are very heat sensitive and should not be heated. This has significant cooking implications.

Avoid omega 6 rich vegetable oils, like canola, sunflower, corn, peanut, safflower, and soybean (several are also GMO—genetically modified) because they increase inflammation (thus heart disease, etc.) Avoid ALL GMO products (most contain the herbicide glyphosate which is harmful). Avoid ALL man-made fats. Even worse than too many omega 6 fatty acids are partially hydrogenated oils or trans fats (e.g., vegetable margarine, Crisco, etc.) You must read the labels and avoid processed food. In short, avoid all man-made fats without any exceptions, which from a practical point of view means avoiding processed foods.

Avoid most fish oil capsules, and instead buy fish or cod liver oil from a known origin. Shrimp may be boiled in salty water, and then you may add avocado mayonnaise or other condiments. Salmon may be "cured" instead of cooked. You may google recipes on line.

A fatty acid profile will determine whether a person has a balanced omega 3 ratio. Zinzino (www.zinzino.com) offers a fatty acid profile home test.

A practical approach is to eat fish or seafood low in mercury (thus avoid large fish like tuna) twice a week. Supplement your oral intake with 5 to 10 ml of high quality fish oil daily.

Dr. Paul Clayton in his book *Out of the Fire* recommends eating fish omega 3, 1-3, 1-6 beta glucans (a prebiotic fiber that reduces inflammation) and polyphenols found in fruits and vegetables. How important they are and whether 1-3, 1-6 beta glucans need to be supplemented is not clear to me.

Fish omega 3 fatty acids are absorbed better if mixed with the polyphenols found in extra virgin olive oil.

1.11. PROTEIN INTAKE.

The ideal diet is high in healthy fats, low or moderate carbohydrates (no refined carbohydrates), and normal protein. Only eat whatever is the amount of protein you need, which is variable and controversial. The recommended dietary allowance (RCA) has been for quite some time 0.8 g per kilogram of body weight (or 0.36 g multiplied by body weight in pounds). Nevertheless, other people have interpreted this recommendation as 0.8 g/kg of lean body weight (body weight minus fat weight). Dr. Gundry, though, recommends 0.37 g of protein per kilogram of body weight/day. The reason for this smaller amount is because he also takes into account the amount of protein recycled daily by the body (about 20 g). Dr. Valter Longo recommends eating 0.31 to 0.36 grams of protein per pound of body weight daily for adults under age 65. https://valterlongo.com/daily-longevity-diet/

In some circumstances protein needs are higher like in infants, children, athletes, and pregnancy, and also in the elderly (age 65 and older) to minimize muscle loss. Most people only need 40 to 70 g/day of protein, at the most. A large amount of protein increases the risk of cancers, decreases the body's pH, and increases the risk of osteoporosis; it will also increase insulin secretion, thus increasing chronic inflammation, which can lead to heart disease, diabetes, and many other chronic degenerative conditions.

Low protein diets have been found to increase longevity in non-elderly adults (higher mortality on a higher protein diet for adults under age 65.[4] In addition, a low protein diet also decreases the risk of dementia in a similar way as calorie restriction. [5]

Ideally, some protein should be from animal origin. It is difficult to eat a complete and well-balanced diet that includes all essential amino acids when eating vegan. B vitamins supplements are also needed when eating vegan. For

---

4 https://www.nih.gov/news-events/nih-research-matters/protein-consumption-linked-longevity and https://www.ncbi.nlm.nih.gov/pubmed/24606898. *Low protein intake is associated with a major reduction in IGF-1, cancer, and overall mortality in the 65 and younger but not older population.* Levine ME -et al. Cell Metab. 2014 Mar 4;19(3):407-17. doi: 10.1016/j.cmet.2014.02.006.

5 http://www.sci-news.com/medicine/low-protein-high-carbohydrate-diet-longevity-06635.html https://www.medicalnewstoday.com/articles/323772.php

this reason, it is a good idea to eat a small percentage of animal protein. Nevertheless, is easier to reverse type 2 diabetes on a pure plant-based diet. One exception might be drinking bone broth and taking a supplement of the nine essential amino acids. Bone broth has a good amount of animal protein with no fat but does not include all essential amino acids. Since insulin resistance is caused by fat not protein, this should be a good compromise. Another option is to take a supplement of whey protein, which includes all essential amino acids.

In their latest book Dr. James Dinicolantonio and Dr. Jason Fung recommend that 50 percent of protein should be from animal origin *(The Longevity Solution)*. I do not think it needs to be this high. I like Dr. Longo's recommendation, mostly plant-based diet and for animal protein only eat fish 2 to 3 times per week, but increase protein intake by 10 to 20 percent at age 65 by adding other products like eggs.

Animal protein should be from healthy sources, like free-range eggs, grass-raised meat (beef, lamb, goat). Feedlot raised animals have been given GMO grains and the animal fat composition changes negatively, so it is no longer healthy for human consumption. Fish should be low in mercury (small fish like sardines, salmon, shrimp, etc), wild caught, NEVER farmed fish, for the same reason.

Too much protein is detrimental. If ingested in a short period, the body will convert some protein into glucose, thus spiking the blood sugar. Animal protein increases acidity (lowers body pH) which is quite harmful if not counteracted by other foods or means (see the book *Alkalize or Die* by Dr. Theodore A. Baroody). Protein stimulates the mTOR gene or pathway, which is good for muscle growth earlier in life but stimulates cancers in general later in adulthood. A more acidic body environment facilitates viral infections, increases osteoporosis, and facilitates cancer growth and spread. Somehow animal products decrease body pH much more than plant-based protein.

1.12. DAIRY PRODUCTS

Dairy products are controversial at best.

Most commercial milk cows produce casein A-1 protein. This specific protein has been associated with many health problems. See *The Plant Paradox* of Dr. Steven Gundry. On the other hand, casein A-2 protein seems to be safe. It is found in the milk of some southern European cows as well as goats.

Goat milk, goat cheese, and sugar-free goat yogurt might be acceptable in small amounts as long as you are not trying to lose weight.

Avoid dairy products if you have prediabetes or type 2 diabetes because insulin sensitivity is worsened by saturated animal fats. Moreover, excess calcium intake will decrease intracellular sodium and potassium, and this will worsens insulin resistance. Excess calcium intake will also increase heart disease risk.

Also avoid dairy products if you are trying to lose weight. All animal proteins stimulate insulin production much more than plant-based protein. A higher insulin level will make it much more difficult to lose weight. Insulin is a hormone that makes the energy stored in fat cells not available. Essentially, insulin locks access to body fat usage.

Animal studies showed increase number of cancers when rats were fed a higher amount of casein. In reality, excess animal protein in general will increase the risk of cancer/s.

It is not true that dairy products are needed to meet daily calcium requirements. In fact, studies in general have not been able to prove that extra milk or calcium supplements decrease the risk of osteoporosis or bone fractures. In at least one study, women eating the largest amount of dairy products suffered more fractures. Enough calcium can be consumed by eating plenty of green leafy vegetables and raw sesame seeds. To prevent osteoporosis, multiple minerals (including magnesium) and trace minerals are needed in the appropriate proportions.

1.13. COOK AT LOW TEMPERATURES.

This is VERY IMPORTANT. It is better not to heat any oils, although coconut oil might be an exception but why to take any chances. Ideally, you should cook without any oils and add oil later. Steaming vegetables is safe. Animal products can be cooked using a Sous Vide water bath or in a crock pot. Using a Sous Vide, meat can be cooked at about between 122 to 140 degrees Fahrenheit or 50 to 60 degrees Celsius. Poultry is usually cooked between 144 and 149 degrees Fahrenheit in a Sous Vide. These are much lower temperatures than traditional ovens.

Avoid cooking food in a way that produces toxic byproducts. Cooking at high temperatures creates the highly harmful AGE's (advanced glycation end products) and ALE's (advanced lipoxidation end products). Both speed up the aging process. Thus avoid or minimize foods grilled, fried, barbequed, or roasted. Avoid deep frying. Foods cooked at no more than 212 degrees Fahrenheit are less prone to AGE/ALE formation. AGE's and ALE's are also found in smoked and cured foods, colas, and powdered milk, thus, avoid them all.

As an example, a sweet potato cooked in the oven is sweeter than when steamed. The higher oven temperature produces more carbohydrates (and sweeter taste) but also harmful AGE's.

1.14. SUPPORT YOUR GUT MICROBIOME AND PREVENT OR REVERSE A "LEAKY GUT."

VERY IMPORTANT. An unhealthy gut microbiome can cause many diseases. The best known microbiome is in the intestines (gut microbiome), which is composed of three different microbiomes: bacteria, viruses, and fungi. The skin also has an important microbiome, although is not as well studied (this is why using daily soap in the shower is a bad idea). Unhealthy food will cause a "leaky gut" (holes in the lining of the intestines) leading to all type of autoimmune conditions and multiple other medical problems like obesity, inflammatory bowel disease, metabolic syndrome, insulin resistance/diabetes, mental and behavioral problems. Avoid all emulsifiers, which are found in many processed foods, because they are not good for the lining of the gut. Examples of emulsifiers are lecithin (often from soy), polysorbate 60 and 80 (made out of petroleum, avoid at any cost), carrageenan, carboxymethylcellulose, xanthan gum, mono- and diglycerides of fatty acids, stearoyl lactylates, sucrose esters, and polyglycerol polyricinoleate. From a practical point of view, the only way to avoid emulsifiers is by not eating processed foods.

Unfortunately, the widely used NSAIDS (non-steroidal anti-inflammatory medications like ibuprofen or naproxen) also disrupt the gut barrier, thus AVOID. Acetaminophen should also be avoided, if possible.

Avoid broad spectrum antibiotics if you can. AVOID GLYPHOSATE because it is an antibiotic that kills the good gut bacteria/microbes. It is the main ingredient of the herbicide Round Up® and most GMO foods come with it. It is also used to spray non-GMO crops before harvesting, thus also avoid by buying organic products.

Your body needs health bacteria supplements/foods (probiotics) and fiber for the bacteria to multiply in the guts (prebiotics). Probiotics in oral form, like sauerkraut, or even enemas are useful. See *Brain Maker* by David Perlmutter, MD. Inulin is a soluble fiber and is a good prebiotic. Other foods with prebiotics include onions, garlic, leeks, Jerusalem artichokes, unripe bananas, yacon, and asparagus. Resistant starches are healthy because they feed gut bacteria, which produce byproducts (short-chain fatty acids like butyrate) used by the colon cells for nutrition. Resistant starches are found in yams, taro, green bananas, shirataki (e.g., Miracle rice or noodles), turnips, beta glucans, legumes, and plantains. Mushrooms also help gut bacteria.

Food products that help in repairing the gut wall include dark berries and grape seed extract. To increase gut bacteria you may also eat sweet potatoes, turnips, parsnips, rutabagas, and a moderate number of figs.

A good review and practical advice on how to prevent or reverse a leaky gut can be found in *Heal Your Leaky Gut* by David Brownstein, MD.

Fecal transplants are very successful treatment for clostridium difficile colitis, also known as pseudomembranous colitis. Many ongoing clinical trials are investigating the potential benefits of fecal transplants for other diseases, including obesity and diabetes.

Control your carbohydrate cravings by completely avoiding sugar and all refined carbohydrates. Gut bacteria communicate with the brain via chemicals and the vagus nerves. Eventually, gut bacteria feeding on these carbohydrates will die out and the cravings will subside. Increased potassium and salt intake might help controlling carbohydrate cravings.

1.15. HYDRATION.

Stay well hydrated by drinking filtered water or tea. Dr. David Brownstein recommends using the following weight/water formula: weight in pounds divided by 2, this is the number of ounces of water needed to stay well hydrated. Caffeinated drinks do not count because caffeine is a diuretic (makes the body lose water).

Do not drink water with fluoride or chlorine. At least three European countries have banned fluoride in potable water because of its potential side effects. The New Zealand Supreme Court ruled that adding fluoride to the water supply is a violation of human rights. The official rationale for adding fluoride to drinking water is to diminish dental cavities. But there is no good evidence to support this practice. In fact, it is considered not helpful but quite dangerous by some experts, like Gerald P. Curatola, DDS. See his book *The Mouth-Body Connection*.

Several ways to filter water are commercially available. The most practical is reverse osmosis which will eliminate fluoride.

Avoid bottled water if possible unless the plastic is BPA free. Glass containers or bottles are ideal.

Tea is very healthy but do not add any sugar. You may add a healthy sweetener like organic liquid stevia or monk fruit. Green tea has more beneficial substances. Brewing tea with boiling water and for longer times might give the tea some bitter taste but the tea will have more medicinal properties.

Coffee is an acceptable drink but remember it can worsen high blood pressure. It can also worsen some irregular heartbeats (like premature ventricular contractions—PVCs). Coffee in moderation does not seem to be harmful.

DO NOT DRINK ANY fruit juices, soda, soft drinks, energy drinks, or sports drinks. They are unhealthy. Sodas with phosphoric acid cause osteoporosis. The no-calorie alternatives are not any healthier and increase obesity and other medical conditions.

1.16. SWEETENERS.

Avoid ALL artificial sweeteners, specifically aspartame (Nutrasweet), sucralose (Splenda), and saccharine. They have too many side effects. Aspartame is a well known neurotoxin (causes nerve damage), even worse when it has been exposed to heat. Do not use in ANY AMOUNT. All these products have been shown to have harmful effects, including increased obesity risk.

Minimize or avoid alcoholic sugars. They can have side effects like a laxative effect, and I am not aware of any long-term safety studies proving their safety. The safest one is erythritol, probably. Xylitol is bactericidal (kills bacteria) and although it has improved gingivitis for some, it is unknown how it will affect gut bacteria in the long-term. If used, buy a non-GMO brand of xylitol (like birch instead of corn) to avoid glyphosate and other pesticides. If you use it, be aware it is fatal to dogs. Maltitol is used in Europe to make sugar-free chocolate, which tastes quite good but quickly causes bloating, flatulence, and diarrhea unless you eat a real small amount. The body does not adapt to maltitol, thus the bloating problem does not improve with time like happens with psyllium (Metamucil).

D-Tagatose is difficult to classify, but it is very similar to alcoholic sugars. Thus, minimize or avoid.

Avoid sweeteners with sugar or fructose. Thus, avoid agave nectar and maple syrup.

Some people think small amounts of honey are acceptable. Maybe this is true but it is mostly sugar. Do not use if you have prediabetes or diabetes because it increases hemoglobin A1c. Never heat honey as it will produce rather toxic byproducts. Heated honey given back to the bees will kill them. In other words, never use honey for baking or cooking if heating is involved.

Yacon might be safe but I doubt most people will like its taste. It can cause excess gas production and diarrhea. It is available in powder form and syrup.

SAFE SWEETENERS include allulose, monk fruit, inulin and stevia. All of them are safe for diabetics. With so many commercially available safe sweeteners, there is no reason why to use an unhealthy one, like sugar. No single safe sweetener works for every recipe. Thus, you will need to figure out how to use them. For example, allulose does not work well for chocolate-making using a melangeur (granite grinder needed to make chocolate). The liquid form is probably the healthiest one since powder sweeteners might have an anticaking agent. Nevertheless, make sure the liquid variety does not have any other ingredients, like natural flavors.

ALLULOSE is D-psicose. It is about 70 percent as sweet as sugar. It can be used for baking. Buy the non-GMO brand. It is available in powder and liquid forms.

MONK FRUIT is 300 times sweeter than sugar. Thus, it might be difficult to use in small amounts. For this reason it often is mixed other products, like erythritol or inulin. It also comes in pure monk powder. It can be used for baking. If you add too much, the final product will not taste as well as expected although it does not have a bitter aftertaste. Pure monk powder is available by several companies: https://www.nunaturals.com/collections/sweeteners/products/monk-fruit-powder

https://julianbakery.com/product/pure-monk-monk-fruit/

https://julianbakery.com/product/pure-monk-usda-organic-pure-monk-fruit-extract-ultra/ (organic version)

https://www.lakanto.com/collections/extract/products/monk-fruit-extract-50-0-71oz https://www.lakanto.com/collections/extract/products/50-0-17-oz

Monk fruit also comes in a liquid form:

https://www.lakanto.com/collections/extract/products/liquid-monkfruit-sweetener-original-flavor and in a chocolate variety https://www.lakanto.com/collections/liquid-sweeteners/products/chocolate-liquid-monkfruit-sweetener

INULIN is a mild sweetener. It is also a prebiotic. A commercially available sweeter product is Just Like Sugar. It does not dissolve as well as allulose. It can be used for baking. In larger amounts can increase gas, bloating, and diarrhea.

STEVIA is also plant-based. It is 300 times sweeter than sugar. Thus, it might be difficult to use in small amounts. For this reason is often mixed with inulin, like in SweetLeaf. It cannot be used for baking (it will lose its sweetness). Some people complain about a mild bitter aftertaste but this is quite variable depending on the brand. I am sure you can find one you like. Cocoa syrup made out of stevia can be used as a sweetener, to make fat bombs or other desserts https://www.nunaturals.com/products/stevia-cocoa-syrup; this specific product tastes very good. Liquid stevia is more convenient because it mixes right away https://sweetleaf.com/stevia_products/sweetleaf-liquid-stevia-sweet-drops/

For an easy fat bomb recipe mix two tablespoons of NuNaturals cocoa syrup (has stevia, no sugar), two tablespoons of very well ground almond butter, two tablespoons of organic cocoa powder, 160 grams of coconut cream, 1/4 teaspoon of liquid vanilla extract, 1/4 teaspoon of cinnamon powder, and a pinch of salt. Place in appropriate container and freeze.

1.17. ADVICE ON CHOLESTEROL AND CHOLESTEROL INTAKE.

Cholesterol is necessary to remain alive. It is in all cells' membranes, is required by neurons, necessary for memory, used to form bile and produce vitamin D and sex hormones, is needed to fight infections, and so on. We could not survive without cholesterol. Most cholesterol in the blood, about 80 percent, is not from dietary intake but produced by the liver. A total cholesterol of less than 160 has been linked to several medical problems including aggression, depression, and decreased sex drive.

Dietary cholesterol/saturated animal fats neither increase "bad" cholesterol in the blood nor cause heart attacks. Let me repeat it. Dietary cholesterol intake DOES NOT GIVE YOU HEART DISEASE. Saturated animal fats do increase total cholesterol and total LDL some but mostly the good LDL (the so called "A particles", which are the larger fluffy ones) and HDL ("good cholesterol"). Total cholesterol and LDL, often used to prescribe statin medications, are not reliable predictors of heart disease. About 50 percent of patients with heart attacks have a normal cholesterol.

To predict heart disease you should use other tests instead, like high sensitive CRP (C-reactive protein), the ratio triglyceride/HDL, particulate LDL, fibrinogen, homocysteine, or a cardiac scan if indicated. A vitamin K2 deficiency increases the risk of heart disease much more than an abnormal total cholesterol and/or LDL (see *Vitamin K2 and the calcium paradox* by Kate Rheaume-Bleue). Also check your vitamin D blood level since low levels correlate with a higher risk of heart disease.

Heart attacks and other degenerative diseases are caused by chronic inflammation not cholesterol intake. Heart disease specifically is mostly caused by chronic inflammation, with other associated risk factors like deficiencies in vitamin K2 and magnesium. Do not confuse vitamin K2 with vitamin K1. The latter one is used for normal coagulation (stop bleeding). Vitamin K1 deficiency is very rare, thus clinically not significant. In Western societies most people are vitamin K2 deficient, though.

The main dietary contributors for heart disease are (a) sugar and (b) "bad fats" (man-made like trans fats and processed vegetables oils) NOT saturated animal fats. Sugar and refined carbohydrates increase triglycerides and this increases chronic arterial inflammation. Triglycerides also increase the small LDL particles (type B). Elevated blood glucose levels also create the very damaging AGEs (advanced glycation end products). Unhealthy fats, like processed vegetable oils or oils heated to high temperatures, will also increase chronic inflammation. A main contributor is a deficiency in vitamin K2 (for more information see www.vitaminK2.org). Vitamin K2, ideally as K-7, improves arterial flexibility, decreases calcium deposits in the arteries, and helps prevent osteoporosis. Vitamin K2 is fat soluble, thus it should be taking with a meal (that includes fat). You may also read *VITAMIN K2: The Missing Nutrient for Heart and Bone Health* by Dennis Goodman, MD, and *VITAMIN K2 AND THE CALCIUM PARADOX* by Kate Rheaume-Bleue, B.Sc., N.D.

Evidence showing saturated fats/cholesterol do not increase heart attacks was already available more than half a century ago in the Framingham Heart Study. The dietary recommendations to decrease saturated animal fats, increase carbohydrates, and increase consumption of processed vegetable oils were due to the research of Ancel Keys, a researcher who had significant ties to the food industry. Several other researchers contradicted him but were quickly "silenced". Ancel Keys studied 21 countries but arbitrarily chose seven to support his hypothesis that coronary artery disease (thus heart attacks) was caused by animal fats. When another researcher used Ancel Keys' data but chose a different group of countries, the culprit were carbohydrates not animal fat. A different researcher re-analyzed the data of all countries to find out animal fat intake did not correlate with heart disease. But there were big financial interests at stake. The food industry benefited by using cheaper processed vegetable oils which have a long shelf life. Heart attacks had become an epidemic during the Ancel Keys years but were caused by smoking, not saturated fats. Ancel Keys' recommendations lead to an excessive intake of refined carbohydrates and processed vegetable oils (and linoleic acid) which increased cancer, cardiovascular disease, and all-cause mortality. Despite the disastrous outcome of Ancel Keys' recommendations, "certain countries exporting this grains would not accept the risks associated with linoleic-rich vegetable oils." [6]

---

6   https://www.karger.com/Article/Pdf/446704 Medicines and Vegetable Oils as Hidden Causes of Cardiovascular Disease and Diabetes. Okuyama H, et al. Pharmacology 2016;98:134–170.

Heart attacks and other degenerative diseases are caused by chronic inflammation. LDL (low density lipoproteins) carries cholesterol to the cells. LDL is only harmful when it has been damaged (oxidized). LDL cholesterol particles when oxidized (from smoking, insecticides, mercury, other toxins, unhealthy fats/oils like omega 6 fatty acids and other foods, etc.) become the small size dense LDL particles (pattern B particles). These small particles end up in the endothelium (inner layer of the arteries) causing inflammation. Only oxidized LDL particles attach to the arterial endothelium. LDL particles are also damaged by high glucose levels. Other causes of increased cholesterol include (a) deficiencies in selenium, iodine, zinc, and copper, (b) chronic infections like gingivitis, (c) elevated cortisol levels due to chronic stress, (d) chronically elevated insulin levels due to insulin resistance and/or eating excessive carbohydrate (decreasing insulin levels can lower cholesterol and blood pressure), and (e) hypothyroidism (low thyroid function).

The body reacts and the immune system attacks the endothelium damaged by the LDL particles with monocytes and macrophages, creating arterial plaque that eventually can block blood flow or rupture and give the patient a heart attack. Once inflammation is detected, the liver increases LDL production to repair tissue damage. The increased cholesterol is an attempt by the liver to correct the inflammatory process (healthy non-oxidized cholesterol is anti-inflammatory). If the LDL particles continue being oxidized (e.g., by tobacco products, stress, unhealthy fats, elevated glucose, etc.) the vicious cycle persists and oxidized small LDL particles will continue damaging the arterial endothelium (inner lining of the arteries). An elevated cholesterol level is a sign of an unresolved underlying abnormality. THERAPY SHOULD BE DIRECTED AT CORRECTING THE UNDERLYING PROBLEM OR CAUSE OF THE DISEASE instead of artificially decreasing cholesterol levels with medications that have side effects.

A couple of examples can clarify this issue. Imagine two towns have the same number of firefighters. In one town few firefighters are working. In the other town multiple ongoing fires require the work of many firefighters. It would make no sense for the mayor of the second town to fire or get rid of a large percentage of firefighters. Instead, the logical approach would be to prevent new fires from starting. If "bad" cholesterol is high, a remedy should be to cure the underlying problem (e.g., smoking, eating sugar or unhealthy fats, etc.) This is why decreasing cholesterol levels with medications, but not curing the underlying cause, is not ideal as it is explained in the statin therapy section.

Another similar example is blowing the smoke away from a house when a nearby fire is rapidly approaching the house. Blowing away the smoke near the house might make the owner feel better but will not help much if the fire is not put out.

Just decreasing cholesterol with medications without correcting the underlying abnormality would be the same as blowing away the smoke or firing the firefighters.

DISSOLVING CALCIUM IN ARTERIES.

Reversing arterial plaque is possible. See protocol for reversal of arterial calcification in SUPPLEMENTS section

10.2.2. ARTERIOSCLEROSIS/ATHEROSCLEROSIS.

CHOLESTEROL THERAPY

BEFORE STATINS. Before statins were commercially available, cholesterol was successfully decreased with other medications but overall survival or heart attack risk did not improve.

STATINS.

Statins are very successful decreasing total cholesterol and LDL. How beneficial they are is more controversial.

Some experts consider statins harmful because they "have been linked to stimulated atherosclerosis and heart failure." [7]

The authors refer to the International Multicenter CONFIRM registry that used CT angiography. Patients on statins had more obstructive coronary disease and the authors concluded "statins accelerate the progression of atherosclerosis" and offered a scientific explanation (statins interfere with the production of vitamin K2). As the reader will find out later, vitamin K2 is critical both for bone and heart health.

Other authors simply conclude "that the expectation that CHD (coronary heart disease) could be prevented or eliminated by simply reducing cholesterol appears unfounded." [8]

7 https://www.karger.com/Article/Pdf/446704, *Medicines and Vegetable Oils as Hidden Causes of Cardiovascular Disease and Diabetes.* Okuyama H, et al. Pharmacology 2016;98:134–170.

8 https://www.ncbi.nlm.nih.gov/pubmed/26225201 Cholesterol confusion and statin controversy. DuBroff R1, de Lorgeril M1. World J Cardiol. 2015 Jul 26;7(7):404-9. doi: 10.4330/wjc.v7.i7.404.

In their comprehensive book review of cholesterol and statins, *The Great Cholesterol Myth*, Drs. J. Bowden and Sinatra recommend statins only for middle age men with known coronary artery disease. They feel statins are contraindicated for the elderly and children, and most women should not use them do to a lack of proven effectiveness but higher risk of side effects (see their book's Chapter Six: *The Statin Scam*). These authors believe benefits from statin therapy are not due to the reduction in cholesterol but to their anti-inflammatory and viscosity reduction properties.

On the other hand, other articles indicate otherwise. A review of other studies showed benefits "in adults at increased CVD risk but without prior CVD events." [9]. Other authors recommend statins for adults 40 to 75 but conclude that "uncertainty exists in those older than 75 years." [10]

Others are willing to recommend statins for primary prevention for the elderly but admit "treatment effects of statins were statistically insignificant in fatal MI (0.43, 0.09 to 2.01), stroke (fatal: 0.76, 0.24 to 2.45; nonfatal: 0.76, 0.53 to 1.11; total: 0.85, 0.68 to 1.06) and all-cause mortality (0.96, 0.88 to 1.04)." [11] The US Preventive Services Task Force specifically excludes starting statins in the elderly "the current evidence is insufficient to assess the balance of benefits and harms of initiating statin use in adults 76 years and older." [12]

Advice on this subject is problematic for several reasons. Often medical experts serving in statin review panels have financial ties or interests with the pharmaceutical industry. Statins are very profitable, thus big profits are at stake. Side effects from statin therapy are quite underreported, thus making difficult to evaluate benefits versus potential complications. In clinical practice, we very often see patients who are "allergic" to one or more statins. In reality, though, it was not an allergic reaction but a medication adverse effect.

In my opinion, appropriate measures should be taken first TO CORRECT THE UNDERLYING CAUSE. This would include quit smoking, avoid all bad fats, avoid processed vegetable oils and heated oils, no sugar or refined carbohydrates. Eat organic. No processed foods. Minimize fructose and no foods with added fructose. Keep the omega 6:3 ratio at 1:1. Exercise. Control stress. Sleep well. Do intermittent fasting (decreases LDL). Take measures as

---

9   https://www.ncbi.nlm.nih.gov/pubmed/27838722

10 https://www.ncbi.nlm.nih.gov/pubmed/28577620

11 https://www.ncbi.nlm.nih.gov/pubmed/26245770

12 https://www.ncbi.nlm.nih.gov/pubmed/27838723

needed to improve insulin sensitivity (see comments in the Diabetes section). Check a fasting insulin level. Elevated insulin levels are highly inflammatory, increase triglycerides, raise blood pressure, increase the risk of obesity and type 2 diabetes mellitus, and increase the risk of coronary artery disease and strokes. Dietary and life style changes are very effective and do not have adverse effects. Wait three months and repeat the appropriate blood work. It is also useful to improve mitochondrial function. This can be done with high intensity interval training (if you are cleared by your provider) and supplements like coenzyme Q10, carnitine, alpha lipoic acid, resveratrol, and vitamin B complex. See supplement section for further details.

Total cholesterol and LDL, often used to prescribe statin medications, are not reliable predictors of heart disease. For this purpose you should use other tests instead, including:

- High sensitive CRP (C-reactive protein), ideal is less than 0.8 mg/L.
- Ratio triglyceride/HDL, ideal is less than 2. It is a significant concern when is > 4.
- Particulate LDL (like the one done in the NMR LipoProfile),
- Fibrinogen, ideal should be less than 400 mg/dL.
- Serum ferritin, should be lower than 80 gm/L.
- Lp(a), normal is less than 30 mg/dL (300 mg/L).
- Homocysteine, which is an independent risk factor value for heart disease. A high level can be treated easily with over the counter B vitamins (B6, B12 and folic acid). The lower the better but should be less than 10 to 12. Anything above 15 is too high.
- Hemoglobin A1c, should be less than 5.7 (5.6 or less) but the lower the better although it has a small J curve when levels are quite low.
- Serum vitamin D level, should be kept on the high normal side.
- ApoB (apolipoprotein B) has a higher predictive value then LDL or total cholesterol. Ideal is less than 100 mg/dL for low or intermediate risk individuals but less than 80 mg/dL for high risk patients.
- And a cardiac scan if indicated. See STUDIES section for further details.

HDL correlates better with heart attacks than total cholesterol or LDL. But HDL also has different particles with good or bad prognosis. The technology to routinely measure these particles is not available yet. HDL level is mostly genetically determined. It can be improved some by physical exercise, omega 3 fatty acids, and a small amount of alcohol (ideally red wine). Some medications not commercially available increased HDL significantly but patients had worse outcomes. Immediate release niacin (vitamin B3) will decrease LDL and triglycerides, as well as increase HDL. The skin flush is not dangerous and stops happening after taking the same dose for a few days. Up to 3,000 mg per day is safe. Recommended dose for this purpose is 500 mg to 2,000 mg per day, starting with a low dose (100 mg/day) and increasing the dose slowly. Dr. Stephen Sinatra recommends up to 4,000 mg per day but it can adversely affect the liver in doses larger than 3,000 mg per day. The other form of vitamin B3, nicotinamide, does not improve cholesterol or triglycerides. Sustained release niacin is more hepatotoxic (toxic to the liver) at 1,500 mg per day and, thus, I would not recommend it unless taking under supervision by a medical provider. Inositol hexaniacinate (or inositol hexanicotinate) is a no flush niacin, still effective in improving cholesterol and triglycerides but more expensive.

The triglyceride/HDL ratio is a much better predictor for heart disease than total cholesterol and/or LDL. The ideal ratio is 2 or less. Greater than four is abnormal and also indicates possible insulin resistance.

Normal fibrinogen levels are between 200 and 400 mg/dL.

An elevated ferritin significantly increases heart attacks, optimal level is below 80 gm/L for women and less than 90 mg/L for men.

Normal A1C is up to 5.6 but a lower number around 5.0 would be better. The higher the A1C, the greater is the risk of developing coronary artery disease.

Many asymptomatic men over age 50 and women over age 65 will have calcium in the coronary arteries. Normal is no calcium at all. A normal coronary calcium scan (cardiac scan) would be reassuring in the presence of abnormal cholesterol numbers. A normal cardiac scan does not have to be repeated for 5 years.

Wait a few weeks before doing a cholesterol/lipid panel after a 5-day fast because fasting temporarily decreases HDL and increases LDL.

A good review can be found in the book Cholesterol Clarity by Jimmy Moore and Eric C. Westmann, MD.

1.18. ALCOHOL.

A 2018 scientific study which included many countries and was published in The Lancet concluded no amount of alcohol is safe. [13] [14] [15]

Alcohol is a leading cause of premature deaths even though some reduction in ischemic heart disease has been observed. [16]

Alcohol is the main cause of liver cirrhosis, a very debilitating fatal disease. Too much alcohol is the main cause of brain atrophy (shrinkage of the brain).

This issue is controversial because many prior studies showed some beneficial effect regarding heart attacks. Alcohol increases HDL, the cholesterol fraction that correlates with fewer heart attacks. Unfortunately, alcohol is a powerful poison and the harmful side effects quickly overshadow any possible benefit. Thus, drink at your own risk and, if you do, in moderation.

If alcohol is consumed, red wine would be the ideal choice. Dr. Gundry has mentioned red wine grown at high altitudes is even healthier. [17]

In their latest 2019 book *The Longevity Solution*, Dr. James Dinicolantonio and Dr. Jason Fung recommend drinking red wine to decrease coronary artery disease. Based on a meta-analysis, the ideal daily alcohol intake is 12.5 grams for women and 25 grams for men. If drinking red wine, this would be about 3 ounces/day for women and 6 ounces/day for men. An older recommendation was two glasses of wine per week for women and 5 glasses of wine per week for men.

Do not drink any alcohol if you are trying to lose weight. People on a ketogenic diet should minimize or avoid alcohol intake. If you do not drink any alcohol, do not start drinking it for the possible health benefits.

1.19. SALT INTAKE.

The ideal amount of salt intake is very controversial. Traditional medical teachings assume the lesser the better but not everybody agrees and extremes are never good.

Excessive intake of salt (sodium chloride) can cause high blood pressure if a person is "salt sensitive". Interestingly, it is the chloride that increases blood pressure. Rats given IV chloride develop hypertension. Sodium without

16 https://www.jwatch.org/fw114508/2018/08/24/alcohol-leading-risk-factor-premature-death

13 https://www.thelancet.com/journals/lancet/article/PIIS0140-6736(18)31310-2/fulltext

14 http://www.euro.who.int/en/health-topics/disease-prevention/alcohol-use/news/news/2018/09/there-is-no-safe-level-of-alcohol,-new-study-confirms

15 https://www.thelancet.com/pdfs/journals/lancet/PIIS0140-6736(18)30134-X.pdf

17 https://www.starnewsonline.com/news/20070319/high-altitude-health

chloride does not increase blood pressure. A good example is sodium bicarbonate, which does not have chloride and does not increase blood pressure. Too much sodium can retain extra fluids, although with normal kidney function sodium is easily lost in the urine.

The solution for hypertension due to excess salt intake is very simple. Avoid too much salt BY NOT EATING ANY PROCESSED FOODS, which are the biggest single source of salt intake. It would be difficult to eat too much salt while eating a plant-based whole food diet cooked at home.

People eating mostly a whole food plant diet can use salt as needed. Avoid the usual "table salt" because it has been bleached, lacks other minerals, and comes with anticaking agents. Instead, buy Mediterranean, Celtic Sea, Himalayan, or Redmond salts because they all have trace minerals which healthy bones need.

Both sodium and chloride are essential, thus necessary for normal life. "Salt sensitive" persons will need to eat less salt to control their blood pressures. The question is whether the person has a real salt sensitivity or has a magnesium and/or potassium deficiency. It is a good idea to do a hair tissue mineral analysis to rule out an intracellular deficiency of magnesium or potassium. It will also determine the intracellular sodium level. A blood level of magnesium is not reliable unless a magnesium RBC test is ordered (magnesium in red blood cells).

If a person's blood pressure is high, the first intervention is to take magnesium and potassium supplements, ideally after doing a hair tissue mineral analysis. Potassium should be taking under medical supervision because there are contraindications, like kidney failure. For example, you may take half a teaspoon of potassium bicarbonate once or twice daily. And you may take ½ to1 teaspoon of magnesium citrate powder every night, or other magnesium you like better (but avoid magnesium oxide due to its poor absorption). It might take a few weeks for the depleted body stores to normalize but should not take that long for the blood pressure to start improving.

As an essential nutrient, salt has benefits. A salt deficiency can increase heart rate, increase weight, increase triglycerides, increase insulin resistance, increase cholesterol, increase peripheral vascular resistance, have a negative effect on cartilage, and increase heart attacks. Based on Dr. James DiNicolantonio, the ideal daily intake of sodium is 3 to 6 grams. One tablespoon of salt (18 grams) has about 7 grams of sodium (this is higher than the official recommended daily allowance). Whether this sodium could be obtained from other sources (e.g., sodium bicarbonate) is something Dr. DiNicolantonio does not specify. See *The Salt Fix* by Dr. James DiNicolantonio.

Salt may also decrease carbohydrate cravings and it will allow most people to enjoy their food and eat more vegetables. The extra magnesium and potassium from the vegetables might counteract any increase in blood pressure caused by salt.

Salt intake losses are increased with profuse sweating, like when using a sauna, thus adjust your daily intake. Nevertheless, the amount of salt lost in sweat decreases significantly when profuse sweating happens on a routine basis.

1.20. BONE BROTH.

Bone broth has many health benefits. It was routinely consumed many decades ago but this tradition has been mostly lost. It should be done with bones from grass-fed or free-ranged animals. Beef bones are simmered (180 to 200 degrees Fahrenheit) 48 hours, chicken bones 24 hours. Chicken feet are good because they have a large amount of collagen. Skin can be used, too.

Chicken bone broth is good for joint cartilage because it has type 2 collagen. Beef bone broth has types 1 and 3 collagen and is good for the skin. For the body to build new cartilage well, at least 500 to 1,000 mg of liposomal vitamin C should be taken twice a day.

At least one study showed homemade bone broth has more collagen then the commercially available. Anyway, grass-fed or free-range commercial bone broth is better than no bone broth at all.

For a complete guide you may read *The Bone Broth Miracle* by Ariane Resnick, CNC.

As expected, not all experts agree. Joel K Kahn, MD, in *The Plant-Based Solution*, advises against drinking animal bone broth because if may contain a small amount of lead. We must balance benefits and risks. I think the benefits in this case clearly outweigh the potential risk. In addition, these are comprehensive guidelines, not to pick and choose but to follow as well as possible. The topic on detoxification will be reviewed later.

1.21. KETOGENIC VERSUS NON-KETOGENIC DIET.

Ketogenic diets have been found to extend life expectancy in mice. [18] An eco ketogenic diet is healthy but not mandatory. It has been shown to improve heart disease risk factors. [19]

---

18 https://www.ncbi.nlm.nih.gov/pubmed/28877457 *A ketogenic diet extends longevity and healthspan in adult mice.* Megan N. Roberts, Cell Metab. 2017 Sep 5; 26(3): 539–546.e5.

A clinical study in 2009 already showed even a short-term eco-Atkins diet (a plant-based ketogenic diet) improved lipid prognostic factors (LDL, total cholesterol/HDL, and apolipoprotein B) compared to a high-carbohydrate diet. LDL dropped more than 20 percent in just two weeks. [20]

The best study available settles this controversial issue beyond any reasonable doubt. It included 85,168 women and 44,548 men followed during 26 years. Deaths were documented in 12,555 women and in 8,678 men. A regular diet was compared to both a low-carbohydrate animal diet and to a low-carbohydrate vegetable diet. Highest all-cause mortality (death rate) was in the low-carbohydrate diet based on animal sources. The vegetable-based low-carbohydrate diet had the lowest all-cause and lowest cardiovascular disease mortality. [21]

As far as I am concerned, the prior study results were predictable because a high percentage of animal products will increase insulin resistance and cancer rates. Of all deaths documented in the study, 41.16 percent (8,740 out of 21,233) were cancer related.

No medical disadvantages or complications from ketogenic diets were found in a 2014 meta-analysis. [22]

In some studies survival has been better on a high carbohydrate diet. How is this possible? Well, this diet would need to have complex carbohydrates mostly from a plant-based diet but without any significant amounts of refined carbohydrates (like bread, pasta, flours, etc.).

---

19 https://bmjopen.bmj.com/content/4/2/e003505 Effect of a 6-month vegan low-carbohydrate ('Eco-Atkins') diet on cardiovascular risk factors and body weight in hyperlipidaemic adults: a randomised controlled trial. Jenkins DJA, et al. BMJ open http://dx.doi.org/10.1136/bmjopen-2013-003505.

20 The effect of a plant-based low-carbohydrate ("Eco-Atkins") diet on body weight and blood lipid concentrations in hyperlipidemic subjects. Jenkins DJ et al. Arch Intern Med. 2009 Jun 8;169(11):1046- 54. doi: 10.1001/archinternmed.2009.115. https://www.ncbi.nlm.nih.gov/pubmed/?term=arch+int+med+2009%3B+169%3A+1046

21 *Low-carbohydrate diets and all-cause and cause-specific mortality: two cohort studies.* Fung TT et al. Ann Intern Med. 2010 Sep 7;153(5):289-98. doi: 10.7326/0003-4819-153-5-201009070-00003. https://www.ncbi.nlm.nih.gov/pubmed/?term=Ann+Intern+Med.+2010%3B+153%3A289

22 https://journals.plos.org/plosone/article?id=10.1371/journal.pone.0100652 *Low Carbohydrate versus Isoenergetic Balanced Diets for Reducing Weight and Cardiovascular Risk: A Systematic Review and Meta-Analysis.* Celeste E. Naude CE et al. PLoS ONE 9(7): e100652. https://doi.org/10.1371/journal.pone.0100652

The body burns fat for energy in a more clean way than carbohydrates. Burning carbohydrates produces more oxygen free radicals, thus speeding up the aging process. In addition, more energy (ATP) is obtained from using fat.

Ketogenic diets are indicated for certain conditions, like children with epilepsy, cancer patients, management of diabetes, and also for weight loss.

Whether a ketogenic diet should be used in patients with type 2 diabetes is controversial because the American Diabetes Association still recommends a fair amount of carbohydrates. Minimizing carbohydrates will make blood glucose control much easier and will decrease the need for medications, like insulin in some cases. Chronic high insulin levels are pro-inflammatory and lead to many complications. The average insulin level will be lower on a ketogenic diet. In fact, some patients might be able to get off their diabetes medications. Keep in mind that saturated animal fats increase insulin resistance, as do man-made fats, processed vegetable oils, and heated fats. Thus, diabetic patients would need to ideally only eat good unheated fats. How much fat is still controversial because low-fat plant-based diets have been very effective in reversing insulin resistance. Please see Diabetes section for more detailed information.

Ketogenic diets are being studied for the treatment of some cancers. [23]

Cancer cells consume a large amount of glucose because they use the anaerobic pathway, which does not use oxygen and yields far fewer calories. The goal of a ketogenic diet is to "deprive" cancer cells from their fuel. Unfortunately, cancer also utilizes glutamine for energy, thus animal protein should be reduced and glutamine inhibitors, like EGCG (epigallocatechin-3-gallate) have been used. Many compounds have been found to also have anticancer properties, like hesperidin, nanoquercetin, quercetin, curcumin, luteolin, baicalein, and tocotrienols. GcMAF activates macrophages and has been effective in the treatment of multiple cancers. [24] Dr. Valter Longo has also shown better response to chemotherapy when fasting is included in the therapeutic regimen.

A ketogenic diet should be low carbohydrates (50 grams or less of net carbohydrates) but normal amount of protein. Some people eat as little as 20 grams of net carbohydrates (total carbohydrates minus grams of fiber). It has also been used by athletes to improve their performance in endurance sports. Ketones will allow them to run longer.

---

23 https://www.mdanderson.org/publications/cancerwise/the-keto-diet-and-cancer—what-patients-should-know.h00-159223356.html

24 https://gcmaf.se/

A ketogenic diet should NOT be high in animal protein as many people think. A high animal protein ketogenic diet is harmful in the long run even though might be helpful to lose weight. Substituting carbohydrates for animal protein and fats increases death rates while substituting carbohydrates for plant protein and fats decreased mortality. [25]

Other researchers have found similar results: "High animal protein intake was positively associated with cardiovascular mortality and high plant protein intake was inversely associated with all-cause and cardiovascular mortality." [26]

It might be even healthier to alternate a healthy ketogenic diet with a non-ketogenic one. Ideally, the body should be able to switch to ketosis. Some people who have been eating a high carbohydrate diet for many years might have a hard time switching to ketosis.

Urine strips can be used to get an idea of how many ketones a person has. Blood tests are much more accurate but the strips are expensive. A non-invasive breath measuring device is commercially available. Ketonix sells a breath ketone analyzer. It is pricey but worth the investment if you are serious about pursuing a ketogenic diet.

Fat bombs can be used to increase percentage fat intake.

An excellent source for ketogenic diets and other helpful health information can be found in a series of videos titled *The Real Skinny on Fat: The Truth about Weight Loss*. It includes 11 episodes and several bonus interviews. This series includes interviews with some of the best experts, it is worthwhile watching. Transcripts are provided with the videos, which were produced by Jeff Hays Films in 2018.

1.22. TYPE 2 DIABETES MELLITUS.

This is a devastating disease, the main cause of blindness, kidney failure, surgical amputations, painful neuropathy, etc. It greatly contributes to heart disease and other cardiovascular problems among many other problems. Prevention is the key.

Type 2 diabetes is usually due to insulin resistance, at least in the earlier stages. Like other degenerative chronic diseases, diabetes is caused by

---

25 https://www.thelancet.com/journals/lanpub/article/PIIS2468-2667(18)30135- X/fulltext.
Dietary carbohydrate intake and mortality: a prospective cohort study and meta-analysis.
Seidelmann SB, et al. THE LANCET V 3, ISSUE 9, PE419-E428, SEPTEMBER 01, 2018.

26 https://jamanetwork.com/journals/jamainternalmedicine/fullarticle/2540540 *Specific-Cause and Cause-Association of Animal and Plant Protein Intake With All Mortality.* Mingyang S. et al. JAMA Intern Med 2016; 176(10): 1463-1453.

epigenetics. In other words, a combination of a genetic predisposition (usually a genetic flaw not well known, and this is why family history is useful to asses risk) and environmental factors. Considering that at least half of the adult population has some degree of insulin resistance, it is clear at least one environmental factor is not known at this time. I speculate it could be pesticides (glyphosate being the worse), other pollutants, heating oils and fats, minerals or trace mineral deficiencies, a vitamin K2 deficiency, or a combination of factors.

Type 2 diabetes is CAUSED BY FAT not sugar (few exceptions might exist). Saturated animal fats are the main culprit or at least are the better studied with more supporting evidence. Other contributing fats are trans fats, man-made fats (e.g., interesterified fats), and processed vegetable oils. Interesterified fats were the worse for glucose control in one study. [27]

Some patients with type 2 diabetes, mostly in later stages, have an autoimmune component that attacks the beta cells in the pancreas. I think this could be secondary to the chronic inflammation caused by high insulin and glucose levels.

Fat as being the cause of diabetes has been proven without a reasonable doubt by a very large body of scientific evidence. It is difficult to understand why so many people, including medical professionals, are not aware of this fact. The first clinical study showing fat as the cause of insulin resistance was done in the early 20th century. The first scientific proof that intracellular fat (increased intramyocellular lipid content in skeletal muscle) was blocking the insulin receptor was published in the *New England Journal of Medicine* in 2004. [28]

Many studies have confirmed those results. MRI technology can be used to detect fat inside the muscle cells. A recent meta-analysis showed polyunsaturated fats (like walnuts, flax seeds or oil, etc.) improve insulin sensitivity and secretion compared to saturated fats, carbohydrates, or monounsaturated fats.[29]

---

27 *Stearic acid-rich interesterified fat and trans-rich fat raise the LDL/HDL ratio and plasma glucose relative to palm olein in humans.* Nutr Metab (Lond). 2007 Jan 15;4:3.
    https://www.ncbi.nlm.nih.gov/pubmed/17224066

28 https://www.ncbi.nlm.nih.gov/pubmed/14960743 *Impaired mitochondrial activity in the insulin-resistant offspring of patients with type 2 diabetes.* Petersen KF1, et al. N Engl J Med. 2004 Feb 12; 350(7):664-71.

29 https://journals.plos.org/plosmedicine/article?id=10.1371/journal.pmed.1002087 *Effects of Saturated Fat, Polyunsaturated Fat, Monounsaturated Fat, and Carbohydrate on Glucose-Insulin Homeostasis: A Systematic Review and Meta-analysis of Randomised Controlled Feeding Trials.* Imamura F et al.

Injection of fat intravenously produces insulin resistance. More saturated fats are found in the blood of insulin resistant patients. And when the fat is removed from the blood, insulin resistance improves.

Nevertheless, other research has shown foods with oleate (like nuts in general, olives, and avocados) also improve insulin sensitivity. In addition, at least one study has shown better insulin sensitivity when carbohydrates are substituted by nonsaturated fats. [30]

All heated fats or oils, even the healthy ones, can cause or worsen type 2 diabetes because they increase insulin resistance. This is probably why in some studies type 2 diabetic patients control their blood sugars quite well on a low fat but high carbohydrate diet (see Dr. Neal Barnard's research).

How heated oils cause diabetes is not well known, at least not at relatively low temperatures. When food is cooked at high temperatures, AGE's (advanced glycation endproducts) are formed which are known to exacerbate insulin resistance. Saturated animal fats are well known to cause diabetes. In a study those participants who ate meat and poultry cooked at high temperatures (like grilled, barbecued, etc.) develop more diabetes then those cooking their meals at lower temperatures, despite eating the same amounts of animal products. [31]

It has been well proven that reusing vegetable oils and deep frying (thus using high temperatures) increases diabetes. When oil reaches its smoke point, it has carcinogens and should be discarded. At what temperature an oil starts becoming unhealthy is not known. Thus, you should cook without any oils. Steaming or boiling (could use bone broth) would be better alternatives. It is not known whether coconut oil is an exemption but in the meantime I would discourage it. Oils can be added after the food is cooked. Better flavor can be obtained by using the right spices or using bone broth which does not have any fat.

A very important question is whether saturated animal fats cause insulin resistance just because they have been heated. Do unheated saturated animal fats cause type 2 diabetes? I cannot find an answer to this question but the answer might be no. In other words, it is possible saturated animal fats cause insulin resistance only when heated. If this is correct, the degree of heat

30 http://care.diabetesjournals.org/content/36/5/1132 *The Effects of Carbohydrate, Unsaturated Fat, and Protein Intake on Measures of Insulin Sensitivity. Results from the OmniHeart Trial.* Gadgil MD et al. Diabetes Care 2013 May; 36(5): 1132-1137.

31 http://care.diabetesjournals.org/content/early/2018/03/05/dc17-1992 *Meat Cooking Methods and Risk of Type 2 Diabetes: Results From Three Prospective Cohort Studies.* Liu G, et al. Diabetes Care 2018 Mar; dc171992.

needed for the fat to become unhealthy is not known. Fats will start blocking the insulin receptor in 150 to 180 minutes. Thus, it would be simple to test this hypothesis. First, eat a good amount of the fat you want to test. Then eat your normal meal. Check blood glucose levels one, two, and three hours after the end of the meal. The 2-hour glucose should be less than 140. The 3- hour glucose should be less than the 2-hour glucose. A 3-hour glucose significantly higher than the 2-hour glucose indicates insulin resistance. Keep on checking hourly glucose levels until they start coming down, to estimate the degree of insulin resistance you suffered. If fat blocked the insulin receptor, the 3-hour glucose will be higher than the 2-hour glucose. I have run this test on multiple occasions and heated fats trigger insulin resistance. For example, four boiled eggs (the tested fat) will significantly increase my 3-hour post meal blood glucose, clearly showing some level of insulin resistance despite my A1c being normal at 5.2 (my lowest was 4.7 on a ketogenic diet). When I eat the same number of eggs, but this time raw eggs, I cannot detect any insulin resistance, not even a minimal elevation of the 3-hour blood sugar. You could do this type of testing at home, using different fats, heated and not heated. But make sure the fat was not heated during the manufacturing process (e.g., ghee is heated and simmered, milk and dairy products are pasteurized, etc.).

Obesity also causes or worsens diabetes by the same fat mechanism. In adulthood people have a mostly stable number of adipocytes (fat cells). Obese persons accumulate much more fat in each adipocyte. This greatly increases the pressure inside the cell, which leaks fatty acids into the blood stream. This fat will also block the insulin receptor.

An excessive amount of sugar or refined carbohydrate can be a contributor to type 2 diabetes. Too much fructose can lead to a fatty liver which causes liver insulin resistance. Refined carbohydrates cause obesity. In other words, carbohydrates can cause type 2 diabetes at least in an indirect way.

Other chemicals have also been linked to insulin resistance.

Multiple deficiencies can cause insulin resistance, including magnesium, chromium, vanadium, copper, omega 3 fatty acids, vitamin D, and others. Supplements for type 2 diabetes include magnesium 400 to 1000 mg daily, vanadium 1 mg with 200 mcg chromium polynicotinate daily (do not buy chromium picolinate), copper 1 mg daily, omega 3 fatty acids (at least 1 gram of DHA + EPA which are the fish oil omega 3), and vitamin D3 (4,000 IU daily).

Interestingly, healthy ketogenic diets improve insulin resistance and this is not just because a smaller amount of carbohydrates are ingested. The explanation is ketones. During a ketogenic diet the body will use ketones for energy. It is thought that ketones themselves improve insulin resistance. [32]

WAYS TO IMPROVE INSULIN RESISTANCE:

Avoid saturated animal fats, unhealthy fats (man-made like margarine, processed vegetable fats) and fats or oils heated to high temperatures. Ideally, fats and oils should not be heated but if you do, cook at the lowest temperature possible. Start a plant-based low fat diet.

It is reasonable to take supplements to treat any deficiencies. Instead of buying every single product, it is convenient to take a multi-ingredient supplement like Nutra-Support Diabetes from Carlson. [33]

The best approach to improve insulin resistance is eliminating the offending factors. Nevertheless, multiple other supplements have been shown to improve insulin sensitivity, including ginger (3 g/day or 3 ginger powder capsules daily if 1 g each), cumin (2 g/day), and cinnamon (½ teaspoon/day). Others include gymnema sylvestre (500 to 1,000 mg daily or 250 mg twice daily), milk thistle extract (1,000 mg daily), African Mango (5,000 mg daily), trans-ferulic acid (500 mg daily), bitter melon (600 mg daily or 50 to 100 ml of juice daily), fish oil (1 to 2 grams daily), DHEA (100 mg daily), vitamin D (4,000 to 5,000 IU daily), alpha lipoic acid (600 to 1,000 mg daily), beta glucans (500 mg daily), resveratrol (1,000 mg daily), polyphenols in cocoa, green tea, and apples.

Other supplements for improving insulin sensitivity or glucose control include turmeric (250 mg of curcumin daily), olive leaf extract, as well as black seed (2 g/day), spirulina (2 to 3 g/day, although up to 19 g/day have been used) [34], ginseng (1 to 3 g/day), and berberine, although the latter is more controversial. Alpha-Cyclodextrin 2,000 mg before meals three times daily has been used both to lose weight and improve blood sugars.

It is not known which one is the best supplement and much less what combination of supplements should be taken. Supplements of potentially deficient minerals should be taken, at least initially. Thus, supplement your diet with magnesium, chromium, vanadium, copper, omega 3 fatty acids. Mineral deficiencies can contribute to diabetes. Nevertheless, mineral supplements will

---

32 https://blog.virtahealth.com/ketogenic-diet-reduce-insulin-resistance/

33 https://www.carlsonlabs.com/nutra-support-diabetes.html

34 https://www.ncbi.nlm.nih.gov/pubmed/12639401 and
https://www.ncbi.nlm.nih.gov/pubmed/30532573

not improve insulin sensitivity unless a mineral deficiency is present. A hair tissue mineral anlaysis might help decide what supplements are needed.

As mentioned above, whether non-heated animal fats increase type 2 diabetes is not known. I have not been able to find a study on how raw unheated animal fats (e.g., raw milk, raw butter) affects insulin sensitivity, and thus type 2 diabetes. It could be that unheated animal fats do not cause diabetes, or maybe increase the risk of diabetes less, but this question remains unanswered. In the meantime, type 2 diabetic patients should avoid saturated animal fats all together.

PRACTICAL APPROACH TO IMPROVING INSULIN RESISTANCE.

Start with a 5-day fast or fast mimicking diet, no animal products. It should be a low fat diet. Dr. Longo's fasting studies have shown improvement of diabetes using periodic 5-day fasts. It is also known that low fat, low calorie diets improve insulin sensitivity. After the 5-day fast, eat raw food for 30 days, including steamed vegetables. It should be low fat (10 percent of caloric intake) diet, without heated oils or heated fats for the reasons mentioned above. Avocados or avocado oil, olive oil, olives, and nuts are allowed (no peanuts or cashews). No roasted nuts or seeds. Still do not eat any animal products. Do not forget to add good quality salt as needed. Avoid all bad fats (processed vegetable oils, man-made fats, saturated animal fats, etc.). Raw nuts (or with some salt) are good but still eat them in moderation. Olive oil and avocado oil are acceptable. May add coconut oil later (still somewhat controversial but there is no scientific evidence showing a problem) but follow blood sugars to confirm it has no negative effect on your blood sugars. Then slowly add other foods while carefully controlling how are they affecting your blood sugars. Do, at least, a fast blood sugar every day as well as a two and three hours post meal blood sugar. The fasting blood sugar should be under 100, the 2-hour under 140 but better if it is < 120. A 3-hour post meal blood sugar will help to decide how much insulin resistance the meal caused.

Some authors feel a higher protein diet helps control blood. It should be mostly plant-based protein. Others studies have found no relationship between protein and insulin sensitivity, though. [35]

It is not clear to me whether protein improves insulin sensitivity or if the improvement is because the pancreas releases more insulin (protein intake releases insulin, animal protein stimulates a higher release of insulin than plant-based protein), thus decreasing blood glucose levels. Probably the latter is correct.

---

35 http://care.diabetesjournals.org/content/36/5/1132 . *The Effects of Carbohydrate, Unsaturated Fat, and Protein Intake on Measures of Insulin Sensitivity. Results from the OmniHeart Trial.* Gadgil MD, et al. Diabetes Care 2013 May; 36(5): 1132-1137.

Just 30 ml of organic apple cider vinegar in a glass of water or tea just before a meal will significantly decrease the post-meal glucose and insulin levels. Do not add any bicarbonate to the vinegar. Other vinegars will work too but organic apple cider vinegar is the first choice.

As mentioned above, cook animal products at the lowest heat possible. I would recommend using water bath (Sous Vide) or a crockpot without any oils. Do not heat any oils.

Start a meal eating veggies and protein, eat carbohydrates afterwards.

Switch to a vegan diet. Even a small amount of fish or meat eaten on a regular basis increases the risk of developing diabetes. A plant-based diet without any animal products has been shown to improve neuropathy pain within a few days, even though the improvement of microscopic nerve damage takes months. This approach has no side effects, something that cannot be said for medications like gabapentin. Of course, on a vegan diet a supplement of vitamin B complex, including B12, is needed.

Minimize caloric intake as much as possible. Instead of daily calorie restriction, you may do intermittent fasting. In a 2014 study, both achieved similar insulin resistance benefits. [36]

A fat-free dressing can be used to decrease total calorie and fat intake. Mix half a cup of coconut aminos with the same amount of organic apple cider vinegar. At the end, add ½ to 1 teaspoon of stevia powder or equivalent amount of liquid stevia (may use monk fruit instead) and a crushed garlic clove. Use this way or simmer for a few minutes until half the volume has evaporated.

Control stress to decrease cortisol levels, which increase blood glucose.

Exercise on a regular basis. It increases the metabolism and improves insulin sensitivity. Aerobic exercise after eating will decrease blood sugar. HIIT (anaerobic exercise) will increase blood glucose (except in type 1 diabetics which should be medically monitored during this type of exercise). This is normal due to gluconeogenesis (new glucose) in the liver. Blood glucose will normalize within 1 to 3 hours.

Lose weight. By losing a few pounds, insulin resistance will improve much. It is not possible to lose weight effectively until blood insulin levels have come down because insulin locks the fat in the body. Low blood insulin levels are very healthy since excess insulin is pro-inflammatory and a great contributor to most chronic degenerative diseases.

---

36 https://www.ncbi.nlm.nih.gov/pubmed/?term=24993615 *Intermittent fasting vs daily calorie restriction for type 2 diabetes prevention: a review of human findings.* Barnosky AR et al. Transl Res. 2014 Oct;164(4):302-11. doi: 10.1016/j.trsl.2014.05.013. Epub 2014 Jun 12.

Insulin resistance test. Measure your blood sugar after eating a specific food product. It should have fat because fat it is the main cause of insulin resistance. Check your blood sugar at 1, 2, and 3 hours. If the 3-hour sugar is as high or higher than the 2-hour sugar, check a 4-hour blood sugar to make sure it is decreasing. Remember, it takes at least 2.5 to 3 hours for fats to negatively affect your insulin receptor. Thus, a 3- or 4-hour blood sugar is a must. When checking to see how a food is affecting your insulin receptor, eat a larger or much larger amount than usual (e.g., three or four times larger) or you might miss a small negative effect.

OTHER SCIENTIFIC SUPPORTING INFORMATION OF TYPE 2 DIABETES BEING MOSTLY CAUSED BY SATURATED ANIMAL FATS

https://ucdintegrativemedicine.com/2016/09/diet-diabetes-saturated-fats-real-enemy/#gs.2rf7yi Diet and Diabetes: Why Saturated Fats Are the Real Enemy.

- The book Dr. Neal Barnard's Program for Reversing Diabetes. By Neal D. Barnard, MD. Rodale 2007.
- The book How Not to Die. By Michael Greger, MD, FACLM.
- https://nutritionfacts.org/2016/11/17/fat-is-the-cause-of-type-2-diabetes/ Fat is the Cause of Type 2 Diabetes. Written By Michael Greger M.D. FACLM on November 17th, 2016

https://nutritionfacts.org/video/what-causes-insulin-resistance/ What causes insulin resistance (saturated animal fat)

1. Arch Intern Med 1927; 40(6): 818-830. Dietary factors that influence the dextrose tolerance test. A preliminary study. S. Sweeney.
2. Diabetology 1999; 42: 113-116. Intramyocellular lipid concentrations are correlated with insulin sensitivity in humans: a 1H NMR spectroscopy study. M. Krssak et al. (diabetes caused specifically by saturated fats).
3. J. Clin. Invest. 1996; 97: 2859-2865. Mechanism of Free Fatty Acid-induced insulin Resistance in Humans. M. Roden, et al.
4. Diabetes 1999; 48(2): 358-64. Rapid Impairment of Skeletal Muscle Glucose Transport/Phosphorylation by Free Fatty Acids in Humans.

5   Metabolism Clinical and Experimental 2013; 62: 417-423. Effects of an overnight lipid infusion on intramyocellular lipid content and insulin sensitivity in African-American versus Caucasian adolescents. S. Lee et al.

6   Diabetes 1999; 48(9): 1836-41. Overnight Lowering of Free Fatty Acids With Acipimox Improves Insulin Resistance and Glucose Tolerance in Obese Diabetic and Nondiabetic Subjects. A TMG Santomauro.

https://nutritionfacts.org/video/the-spillover-effect-links-obesity-to-diabetes/
The Spillover Effect Links Obesity to Diabetes

1   News Physiol Sci 2004; 19: 92-96. How Free Fatty Acids Inhibit Glucose Utilization in Human Skeletal Muscle. Michael Roden.

2   Diabetes 2001; 50: 2579-2584. Effects of Intravenous and Dietary Lipid Challenge on Intramyocellular Lipid Content and the Relation With Insulin Sensitivity in Humans. Oliver P. Bachmann, et al.

https://nutritionfacts.org/video/lipotoxicity-how-saturated-fat-raises-blood-sugar/ Lipotoxicity: How Saturated Fat Raises Blood Sugar

1   Cell 148, March 2, 2012. *Mechanisms for Insulin Resistance: Common Threads and Missing Links.* Vaman T Samuel et al.

2   Progress in Molecular Biology and Translational Science, Volume 121. *Free Fatty Acids and Skeletal Muscle Insulin Resistance.* Lyudmila I. Rachek **(insulin resintance caused by saturated fats, not by unsaturated fats).**

3   JAMA Intern Med 2013; 173(14): 1335-1336. *Oxygen-Carrying Proteins in Meat and Risk of Diabetes Mellitus.* William J. Evans **(saturated fats cause insulin resistance).**

4   Diabetes Vol 48, August 1999. *Intramyocellular Triglyceride Content Is a Determinant of in Vivo Insulin Resistance in Humans.* Gianluca Perseghin, et al. **(saturated fat build up in muscles causes insulin resistance).**

5   Journal of Gastroenterology and Hepatology 2009; 24: 703-711. *Lipotoxicity: Why do saturated fatty acids cause and monounsaturated protect against it?* Christopher J. Nolan et al. **(saturated fats cause lipotoxicity).**

6   Endocrine, Metabolic & Immune Disorders – Drug Targets
     2007; 7: 65-74. *Role of Insulin in the Pathogenesis of Free Fatty
     Acid-Induced Insulin Resistance in Skeletal Muscle.* Jianping Ye
     (insulin creates free fatty acid insulin resistance).

7   Mediators of Inflammation 2013; article ID 13. *Lipotoxicity:
     Effects of Dietary Saturated and Transfatty Acids.* Debora
     Estadella, et al. **(saturated and trans fatty acids cause insulin
     resistance).**

8   Diabetologia 2001; 44: 312-319. *Substituting dietary saturated
     for monounsaturated fat impairs insulin sensitivity in healthy men
     and women: The KANWU study.* B Vessby, et al. **(insulin
     sensitivity improved by switching from saturated fats to
     plant fats: insulin sensitivity was impaired on saturated fat
     but not on monounsaturated fatty acid diet-olive fat).**

9   Lipids in Health and Disease 2012; 11: 30. *Mechanisms
     underlying skeletal muscle insulin resistance induced by fatty acids:
     importance of the mitochondrial function.* Amanda R Martins, et al.
     **(saturated fats cause insulin resistance – e.g., palmitic acid
     and stearic acid are potent inducers of insulin resistance
     also inhibit key mitochondrial enzymes).**

10   Annals of Nutrition & Metabolism 2008; 53: 29-32. *Vegetarian
     Diet Affects Genes of Oxidative Metabolism and Collagen Synthesis.*
     Heidrun Karlic, et al. **(on a vegetarian diet have 60 percent
     higher expression of fat burning enzyme).**

11   European Journal of Clinical Nutrition 2005; 59: 291-298.
     *Veganism and its relationship with insulin resistance and
     intramyocellular lipid.* LM Goff et al. **(vegans had lower
     systolic blood pressure, higher intake of carbohydrates;
     vegans had less fat in muscle despite having same BMIs).**

12   European Journal of Clinical Nutrition 2013; 1310-1315.
     *Higher insulin sensitivity in vegans is not associated with higher
     mitochondrial density.* J Gojda, et al. **(vegans had better insulin
     sensitivity, better blood glucose levels, better insulin
     levels, and higher insulin glucose disposal, as well as
     improve beta cell function. Thus, veganism is
     cardioprotective and possible beta cell protective).**

https://nutritionfacts.org/video/plant-based-diets-and-diabetes/ Plant-Based Diets & Diabetes

1   Diabetes 1971; 20: 99-108, February. *Influence of Nutritional Factors on Prevalence of Diabetes.* Kelly M West, et al. **(animal fat consumption was positively associated with diabetes prevalence).**

2   Am J Public Health 1985; 75: 507-512. *Does a Vegetarian Diet Reduce the Occurrence of Diabetes?* David A Snowdon, et al. **(eating meat one or more day a week increases the risk of diabetes; risk increases with increased number of days meat was eaten, despite controlling for weight; lower prevalence of diabetes among vegetarians).**

3   Nutrition, Metabolism & Cardiovascular Diseases 2013; 23: 292-299. *Vegetarian diets and incidence of diabetes in the Adventist Health Study-2.* S Tonstad, et al. **(diabetes decreases with the level of vegetarian diet: 0.22 for vegans, 0.39 for lactoovovegetarian, 0.49 for pescovegetarian, 0.72 for semivegetarian. N = 89,224 individuals. Same applicable to high blood pressure and BMI).**

4   PLoS 2014 February 11; 9(2): e88547. *Taiwanese Vegetarians and Omnivores: Dietary Composition, Prevalence of Diabetes and IFG.* Tina H T Chiu, et al. (vegetarian compared to traditional Asian diet with a very small amount of animal products **(women ate a single serving per week, men every few days): men eating vegetarian had half the rate—0.49—of diabetes and 0.66 for IFG; in pre-menopausal women: diabetes 0.26 and IFG 0.60; and in menopausal women: diabetes 0.25 and IFG 0.73. IFG = pre-diabetes = impaired fasting glucose. No analysis done between vegetarian and vegan but there were no cases of diabetes among vegans).**

https://nutritionfacts.org/video/what-causes-diabetes/ What Causes Diabetes?

1   Mediators of Inflammation 2013; article ID 13. *Lipotoxicity: Effects of Dietary Saturated and Transfatty Acids.* Debora Estadella, et al. **(saturated and transfatty acids can destroy beta cells).**

2   Diabetes 2012; 61: 2763-2775. *Death Protein 5 and p53-Upregulated Modulator of Apoptosis Mediate the Endoplasmic Reticulum Stress—Mitochondrial Dialog Triggering Lipotoxic Rodent and Human beta cell Apoptosis.* Daniel A. Cunha, et al. **(mostly saturated fat (palmitate) negatively affects beta cells; olives, nuts and avocados (oleate) has a minimally negative effect).**

3   Biochemical Society Transactions 2008; volume 36, part 3. *Fatty acids and glucolipotoxicity in the pathogenesis of Type 2 diabetes.* **(LDL can cause beta cell death; increased level of free fatty acids impair pancreatic beta cell function in vivo).**

4   Diabetologia 2006; 49: 1371-1379. *Differential effects of monounsaturated, polyunsaturated and saturated fat ingestion on glucose-stimulated insulin secretion, sensitivity and clearance in overweight and obese, non-diabetic humans.* C. Xiao, et al. **(saturated fat negatively affects insulin secretion and function; increased insulin resistance and decreased insulin production within hours of saturated fat ingestion).**

5   JAMA Intern Med 2013; 173 (14): 1335-1336. *Oxygen-Carrying Proteins in Meat and Risk of Diabetes Mellitus.* William J. Evans **(red meat consumption increases diabetes risk).**

6   Dig Dis Sci 2014; February 59(2): 346-57. *Saturated Free Fatty Acid Sodium Palmitate-Induced Lipoapoptosis by Targeting Glycogen Synthase Kinase-3B Activation in Human Liver Cells* **(fat—e.g., palmitate—in meat and dairy are universally toxic; fat in nuts and avocados (monounsaturated fatty acids—MUFA—e.g., oleat—are not toxic).**

7   Progress in Lipid Research 2013; 52: 165-174. *Molecular mechanisms and the role of saturated fatty acids in the progression of non-alcoholic fatty liver disease.* Alexander K Leamy, et al. **(saturated fat is toxic to liver cells; plant fat is not toxic).**

8   Am J Clin Nutr 1993; 58: 129-36. *Relationship of dietary saturated fatty acids and body habitus to serum insulin concentrations: the Normative Aging Study.* Donna R Parker, et al. **(obesity and saturated fat intake increase fasting and postprandrial insulin concentrations).**

9   Circulation 1991; 84: 2020-2027. *Saturated Fat Intake and Insulin Resistance in Men With Coronary Artery Disease.* David J. Maron **(saturated fat as a contributor to insulin resistance).**

10   Am J Clin Nutr 2003; 78: 91-8. *Plasma fatty acid composition and incidence of diabetes in middle-aged adults: the Atherosclerosis Risk in Communities (ARIC) Study.* Lu Wang, et al. **(increased plasma saturated fatty acids increased the risk of diabetes).**

11   Diabetologia 2008; 51: 1781-1789. *Pathogenesis of type 2 diabetes: tracing the reverse route from cure to cause.* R. Taylor **(diabetes is caused by the consumption of too many calories rich in saturated fats).**

https://nutritionfacts.org/video/why-is-meat-a-risk-factor-for-diabetes/
Why Is Meat a Risk Factor for Diabetes?

1   Curr Diab Rep 2013 April; 13(2): 298-306. *Meat Consumption, Diabetes, and Its Complications* **s**

2   Diabetologia 2013; 56: 47-59. *Association between dietary meat consumption and incident type 2 diabetes: the EPIC-InterAct study. The InterAct Consortium* **(meat consumption increased risk of diabetes; also seen an increase risk of diabetes among workers in the meat industry, unclear cause).**

3   Nature Reviews Molecular Biology January 2011; volume 12. *mTor: from growth signal integration to cancer, diabetes and ageing.* Roberto Zoncu, et al. **(excessive animal/dairy protein/food consumption over stimulates mTor and may increase diabetes due to increase intake of leucine)**

4   World J Diabetes 2012; March 15, 2012; 3(3): 38-53. *Leucine signaling in the pathogenesis of type 2 diabetes and obesity.* Bodo C. Melnik **(large amount of leucine only in animal protein).**

5   Alternative Therapies Mar/April 2010; volume 16, No 2. *Environmental toxins, obesity, and diabetes: an emerging risk factor.* Mark A. Hyman **(organic pollutants and heavy metals as contributors to obesity and diabetes).**

6   Diabetes & Metabolism 2014; 40: 1-14. *Persistent organic pollutants and diabetes: A review of the epidemiological evidence.* D.J. Magliano, et al. **(main source of organic pollutants is intake of dietary intake of animal fats).**

https://nutritionfacts.org/video/how-to-prevent-prediabetes-from-turning-into-diabetes/ How to Prevent Prediabetes from Turning into Diabetes

1   Non drug approaches (life style modifications) are superior to medications (Metformin) to prevent diabetes.

2   No patients with prediabetes who follow the guidelines and met their goals developed diabetes: N Engl J Med 2001; 344(18) Jaakko Tuomilehto et al.

https://nutritionfacts.org/video/preventing-prediabetes-by-eating-more/ Preventing Prediabetes by Eating More

1   Archives of Iranian Medicine Sept 2012; 15(9). *Legume Intake is Inversely Associated with Metabolic Syndrome in Adults.* Somayeh Hosseinpour-Niazi, et al. **(decreased risk of prediabetes by eating more legumes)**

2   British Journal of Nutrition 2012; 108, S111-S122. *Regular consumption of pulses for 8 weeks reduces metabolic syndrome risk factors in overweight and obese adults.* R. C. Mollard, et al. **(pulses = legumes; compared beans ad libitum—5 cups/week—vs. caloric restriction; bean group reduced prediabetes factors— e.g., better blood glucose control).**

1.23. OBESITY

FAT DOES NOT MAKE YOU FAT, refined carbohydrates do. Obesity is a very complex problem because it can be due to many different conditions or factors. It has a large genetic component. But in most cases also requires environmental factors. Delivery by C-section significantly increases its risk as does the lack of maternal breast feeding. A vaginal delivery allows the baby to get healthy vaginal bacteria that will colonize the gut and help the infant's microbiome. The same happens with breast feedings. Breast milk has healthy bacteria.

You should rule out endocrine (e.g., low thyroid function, insulin resistance) and toxic conditions (e.g., mercury intoxication), if none is found start a plant-based ketogenic diet. You should know your fasting insulin level. If your fasting insulin level is high (ideal is less than 5), then you must bring it down or the elevated insulin will lock the fat in place.

Initially, avoid all animal products and alcohol. Avoid saturated fats in general. The exceptions are coconut oil and MCT (medium chain triglycerides). Avoid all unhealthy oils, the body will store them in the adipocytes (fat cells)

but will not know how to use them to produce energy. This will make losing weight very difficult. You should have a home glucometer and find out how specific meals are affecting your 2-hour and 3-hour post meal blood sugar (glucose). This is VERY IMPORTANT and it should be done by every adult even if not obese.

Both fasting and intermittent fasting (restricted feedings) will help when trying to lose weight. In one study, weight loss was not as pronounced with restricted feeding/intermittent fasting as with caloric restriction but the latter is more difficult to implement and follow on a chronic basis. Some type of fasting or restricted feeding should be an integral part of a weight loss program. Besides being helpful to lose weight, fasting has many health benefits.

If you still do not lose weight, further medical work up to rule various conditions is indicated (e.g., decreased thyroid function, food allergies/sensitivities, low testosterone, increased inflammation, mineral deficiencies, excessive chronic stress, female hormones imbalance, heavy metal poisoning, and so on). For the work up of medical conditions see *The Blood Sugar Solution* by Dr. Mark Hyman.

If a ketogenic diet fails, you could try the Plan Z diet (https://www.planz-diet.com/) which uses a spray four times a day to control hunger cravings. Another option is the HCG (human chorionic gonadotropin) diet, ideally using injections not oral medication. The HCG diet works by increasing anabolic hormones.

A way to follow your progress is not just checking your weight but also using a fat caliper (see *The Blood Code* by Dr. Richard Maurer for further details).

IF everything fails:

Consider switching temporarily to a ketogenic diet high in animal protein because it suppresses appetite. Two concerns with this diet. First, animal fats can increase insulin resistance. Thus, you should use a glucometer to make sure your blood sugars do not start rising. A two or three hour post meal blood sugar will inform you whether a meal should be avoided. Do not eat that food if your 2-hour sugar is 140 or higher, and/or the 3-hour blood glucose is significantly higher than the 2-hour glucose. Second, the other problem is long-term complications. As soon as you have achieved your ideal weight you should switch to a mostly plant-based diet as described in these guidelines.

A WORD OF CAUTION. The degree of toxic products accumulated in the human body is very high. Many toxins are liposoluble (they dissolve in fat) and, thus, accumulate in the adipose (fat) tissue. Among these toxic products are toxic metals and persistent organic pollutants. When losing weight, these toxins will be released and may cause major side effects. In addition, toxins released during weight loss might be a major contributor to regaining the lost weight. For a detailed explanation the reader is encouraged to read *Ketofast* by Dr. Joseph Mercola. My advice is to always start a detoxification protocol while losing weight. You should at least do the HIIT + infrared sauna protocol during a weight loss program (see below).

2. FASTING. CALORIE RESTRICTED DIET VS. FASTING.

VERY IMPORTANT. Fasting is one of the most effective ways to remain healthy. It does not take any time and is free. No sophisticated knowledge is needed.

Excess calorie intake speeds up aging. Food is metabolized into energy and this process produces free radicals which damage the cells and their organelle. Carbohydrates produce more free radicals. Fats (e.g., ketones) burn more cleanly, thus they are a better and healthier energy source for the human body.

Periods of fasting are very healthy. Fasting is included in all major world religions and is becoming better studied and understood. It should be an integral part of healthy habits.

One oncology study showed improved immune system function with a 3-day fast. Fasting is a must when trying to lose weight or reverse chronic degenerative conditions. Multiple techniques have been described and there are no good studies to prove which one is the best option.

Fasting should not be confused with what many people call "intermittent fasting" which actually is restricted feedings. Fasting implies a minimal of 24 hours without food intake, some experts think this time period should be longer (like 1.5 to 2 days) to be real fasting. The so called "intermittent fasting" is a form of restricted eating, usually not eating anything for at least 16 hours a day. In other words, all food intake happens within a few hours, traditionally 8 hours although shorter time periods might be better. Intermittent fasting (restricted feedings) will not increase the number of circulating stem cells but offers many health benefits, like decreased risk of heart disease, atherosclerosis, hypertension, obesity, and type 2 diabetes. It is clear that the old recommendation of eating six meals a day (thus all day long) cannot be supported by current scientific evidence. A recent review of "intermittent fasting" can be found at https://www.ncbi.nlm.nih.gov/pmc/articles/PMC6471315/ [37]

---

37 *Intermittent Fasting in Cardiovascular Disorders–An Overview.* Malinowski B et al. Nutrients. 2019 Mar; 11(3): 673. Published online 2019 Mar 20. doi: 10.3390/nu11030673

To make matters more complicated and confusing, people also use the term "intermittent fasting" for real intermittent fasting. The most popular protocol is the 5:2 diet. In short, it is 5 days without any caloric restrictions, then two days eating about 500 calories per day. Any type of fasting will have benefits and this one is not an exception. It should decrease heart disease, strokes, and help weight loss. [38]

MY ADVICE ON FASTING. An excellent approach to fasting is a two-prong system which entails doing two types of fasting:

1. First, do "intermittent fasting" (restricted feedings). A practical way is based on the circadian rhythm, thus eating all meals within a 4 to 6 hour period. What time of the day is debatable. Some experts think earlier in the day is best. I think later in the day is easier to follow, as long as food intake finishes at least three hours before going to bed. The shorter the eating period, the healthier it is because it will improve insulin resistance more effectively. Nevertheless, some foods (healthy fats) can be ingested during the fasting period without breaking the fast, as long as they do not have any protein or carbohydrates. For example, a salad with spinach and avocado mayonnaise that contains no protein or carbohydrates; or spinach with coconut oil, or with olive oil and vinegar/salt. Or a few olives. Another option is to eat a salad of vegetables, like celery, cabbage, red cabbage, sauerkraut, and leafy greens using a fat-free dressing (see one delicious recipe below). Of course, products without any significant calories like broth, green tea, water, etc., will not break the fast. Good information can be found in *The Obesity Code* by Dr. Jason Fung and *Ketofast* by Dr. Joseph Mercola.

2. Second, 5-day fast or a 5-day fast mimicking diet. Both restricted feedings and 5-day fasts can be combined for better results. In other words, restricted feedings and fasting are not exclusive. The 5-day fast will stimulate the body to introduce into circulation stem cells which rejuvenate the body. Stem cells are released after 3 days of fasting. For more details read *The Longevity Diet* from

---

38 *Intermittent v. continuous energy restriction: differential effects on postprandial glucose and lipid metabolism following matched weight loss in overweight/obese participants. Br J Nutrition* Volume 119, Issue 5,14 March 2018, pp. 507-516. https://www.cambridge.org/core/journals/british-journal-of-nutrition/article/intermittent-v-continuous-energy-restriction-differential-effects -on-postprandial-glucose-and-lipid-metabolism-following-matched-weight-loss-in-overweightobese-participants/B165A5BA52A6B625B7A98067D3B2F39B

Valter Longo, Ph.D. Dr. Longe promotes a 5-day mimicking diet because it is easier to do while having the same benefits as water fasting. What to eat those 5 days can be found on several web pages. Prepackaged food is also commercially available at https://prolonfmd.com/ How often to do a 5-day fast depends on multiple variables. A healthy young adult at about age 30, might only need to do it once a year. An adult with significant chronic medical conditions will benefit from doing a 5-day fast once a month. Another alternative is to fast as defined by other researchers, e.g., less than 400 calories/day. It should be mostly green leafy vegetables with some healthy fats like olives but minimal or no protein.

One great benefit from fasting is autophagy. This means the cells recycle old components, protein, and organelles. Autophagy is very health and prevents chronic conditions and cancers. Be careful because autophagy will stop once a person starts ingesting a significant amount of protein. Also 5-day fasting will lead to apoptosis, where unhealthy cells will die out before turning into cancer cells.

After having done many 5-day fasts, using the main techniques, I think the easiest one to do is less than 400 calories per day, eating only vegetables like celery, spinach, cabbage, red cabbage, kale, sauerkraut, or similar vegetables (no root vegetables), and even a small amount of mushrooms. For salad dressing, you may use the fat-free dressing described above that uses coconut aminos and organic apple cider vinegar. A small amount of plant-based fat, like green olives, is acceptable. You can eat a large amount of food if you follow this guideline. For illustrative purpose, to follow are calories in 100 grams (3.5 ounces) of vegetables: celery: 16; red cabbage: 31; cabbage: 26; sauerkraut: 27; spinach: 23; and mushrooms: 22. Mushrooms have the highest protein content (3.3 grams per 100 grams), thus do not eat a large amount while fasting.

Pure water fasting is difficult for most people and you would need to ingest some salt (e.g., broth or similar).

Whether supplements, like minerals and vitamins, should be taking during a 5-day fast is controversial. One study showed better results when taken but other experts disagree. Some supplements stop autophagy, like vitamins C and E, and NAC (N-Acetylcysteine). Autophagy is stimulated by fasting, berberine, lithium, glucosamine, and resveratrol.

Cycles of a 5-day fast mimicking diet have been scientifically found to improve risk factors for aging and age-related chronic conditions, including diabetes. [39]

Contraindication to fasting include:

- malnourishment,
- very low body weight (BMI < 18.5), which is very unusual and a medical work up is probably indicated,
- pregnancy and breastfeeding.
- Valter Longo does not recommend it after age 65 but this is debatable.

Two good sources for fasting information are *Ketofast* by Dr. Joseph Mercola and *The Complete Guide to Fasting: Heal Your Body Through Intermittent, Alternate-Day, and Extended Fasting* by Dr. Jason Fung.

3. EXERCISE

Physical activity is a must. The best exercise is HIIT (high intensity interval training).

Thus, avoid sedentary life. Exercise decreases insulin resistance and inflammation. As mentioned, the best exercise is high intensity interval training (HIIT), which can be done in 16 to 18 minutes, 3 to 4 times weekly (hopefully no less than twice weekly). Exercise while fasting is acceptable, in fact it might be more beneficial, but could be contraindicated and requires medical supervision in diabetic patients who take diabetic medications.

Exercise helps blood sugar control. Nevertheless, strenuous exercise will briefly increase blood sugars in non-diabetic persons but this does not pose any harmful side effects and usually blood sugars return to normal within one to three hours.

Example of an HIIT exercise on a stationary bicycle. Check with your physician or medical provider to make sure you are fit for this type of physical activity. First minute do aerobic pedaling. This means exercising at about 70 to 75 percent of your maximum heart rate. You may Google your maximum heart rate because it decreases with increasing age. Then do 20 seconds of anaerobic pedaling at about 85 to 90 percent of maximum heart rate, which can be summarized as fast as you can. Use some type of monitor, like a step-counting watch or a pulse oximeter placed on the tip of one finger, at least the first few times until you figure out your biking speeds. Repeat several times for

39 https://www.ncbi.nlm.nih.gov/pubmed/28202779

about 16 minutes. In short, start aerobic exercise at minutes 0', 1'20", 3'40", 6', 8'20", 10'40", and 13'. Start the 20-second anaerobic exercises at 1', 3'20", 5'40", 8', 10'20", 12'40", and 15'.

Resistance training (e.g., weight lifting and similar exercises) is also very good. It is ideal to maintain or increase muscle mass. Thus, it is very helpful for older people who should try to at least maintain their muscle strength. Aerobic exercise will not prevent muscle mass decline. Taking 10 to 20 grams of protein just before or after exercising will help muscle buildup (see P.D. Mangan's book *Best Supplements For Men*, which for this purpose is applicable to women also). Adam Zickerman recommends slow motion exercises (10 seconds lifting and 10 seconds lowering), which should decrease or prevent injuries.

A WORD OF CAUTION. Exercise alone without other lifestyle changes, like healthy foods, will not suffice. It will not prevent chronic degenerative conditions, like heart disease.

4. CONTROL CHRONIC STRESS

Chronic stress is very harmful because increases cortisol levels (a stress hormone produced by the adrenal glands). It will also decrease intracellular magnesium (used to metabolize stress hormones), which is necessary for energy production in the mitochondria. Several techniques are available to control stress, including meditation, yoga, Reiki, saunas, etc. In the long-term, chronic stress will lead to many chronic medical conditions, including heart attacks. High levels of cortisol negatively impact the whole body, including the immune system, and have been shown to increase hypertension, cancers, and many other diseases.

Meditation is the most effective way to control stress. Just 5 to 10 minutes daily will suffice although it can be increased to 15 to 20 minutes. You may concentrate on your breathing and disregard the random thoughts which unavoidably will happen. To increase the beneficial effect of meditation by taking advantage of Earth's magnetic field, you should meditate facing the magnetic North Pole. Meditation will be even more effective if you place a magnet on your forehead (place two round magnets on the inside and outside of a head band to keep them together). The north pole of the magnet should be facing Earth's magnetic North Pole. You can use two magnets placed on each side of a headband or just one magnet in a commercially available headband. A magnet that holds at least one pound (half a kilogram) is enough. Neodymium magnets are the best (no reason why to use any other type of magnet). Meditation done this way increases the vibrational frequency of the quantum energy a person has, the so-called "soul" or "aura" by others. I have to delegate to quantum physics experts to understand how this happens. A higher quantum energy in the brain can help cure or at least ameliorate physical conditions. Another reason to be positive and happy, thinking the glass is half full not half empty.

At least one study showed a larger decrease of inflammatory markers with meditation compared to deep breathing exercises.

Other stress control techniques include Reiki, yoga, listening to relaxing music, and deep breathing exercises.

Control stress at work. Working should be a way for you to do what you like and are passionate about, not to destroy your health. If you do not like your current job, switch to something you enjoy doing. Life is too short to be working in a job you do not like. Your work should be one of your hobbies not just a way to get a pay check. If you are a retiree, do not try to accomplish too many projects because it will increase your stress level.

Sleep 8 hours per day. Do not be sleep deprived; most people need to sleep 8 hours/day. Try to sleep at about the same time every day. Chronic lack of sleep is very harmful, leading to many conditions like high blood pressure, worsening insulin resistance, obesity, etc.

5. AVOID TOXINS AND DETOXIFY

5.1 AVOID ENVIRONMENTAL TOXINS.

Avoid exposure to any pesticides. Insecticides, for example, increase neurological diseases like Parkinson's disease. If you have a garden or a lawn, use organic products not petroleum-based fertilizers and pesticides. Thus, do not use Round Up®. Use alternative organic methods to get rid of weeds.

Clean or replace furnace filters frequently. Hopefully you do not live by a highway where car pollution unavoidably will reach your house. Clear air ducts in your home. A HEPA filter to clean the air is helpful if the house is not too big.

Avoid most household cleaners. If you can smell them, they are negatively affecting your body. People with autoimmune problems, like multiple sclerosis, should be very careful with any man-made chemicals.

Use organic laundry detergent. Avoid all harsh chemicals.

5.2. COOKING HARDWARD AND FOOD STORAGE.

Avoid aluminum, teflon/non-stick, copper cookware. Use stainless steel, granite coated, ceramic, or ceramic-coated cookware. Ceramic cookware is expensive and has to be heated slowly.

Store food and liquids in glass containers to avoid plastic/BPA. Many food cans have plastic lining that has BPA. Place vegetables just purchased in cotton bags as soon as you get home. Then place the cotton bag in a plastic bag to keep the moisture in.

Also avoid aluminum containers.

Avoid toxic chemicals like fluoride, deodorants with aluminum, etc.; thus, only use organic cosmetics, toothpaste, deodorants, etc. To avoid fluoride you may use reverse osmosis to purify your drinking water.

5.3. DEODORANTS

Avoid deodorants with unhealthy products, like aluminum which has been shown to increase breast cancer in the upper outer quadrant when those deodorants with aluminum are used. You could make your own deodorant. Lime or lemon juice will work. Or make a paste by mixing sodium bicarbonate (baking soda) with coconut oil. Safe commercial deodorants are available, like Love Myself organic. [40] [41] [42] [43]

5.4. ORAL HYGIENE

Good oral hygiene is important to decrease the risk of heart disease. Chronic gingivitis (inflammation or swelling of the gums) increases the risk of heart attacks. Use a healthy fluoride-free toothpaste. See The Mouth-Body Connection by Gerald P. Curatola, DDS. Revitin is a good prebiotic toothpaste which will help if you have any degree of gingivitis. [44] In his book Dr. Curatola gives a recipe to make your own healthy toothpaste at home.

5.5. SKIN PRODUCTS.

Always use organic products. The rule of thumb of what can you apply to your skin is simple: Do not use it if you are not willing to eat it.

---

40 https://www.amazon.com/Green-Tidings-Organic-Deodorant-Unscented/dp/B00EOB000Q?th=1

41 https://www.amazon.com/gp/product/B007BUKB4C/ref=ppxyodtbsearchasin title?ie=UTF8&psc=1

42 https://www.amazon.com/gp/product/B01E3D2CEG/ref=ppxyodtbsearchasin title?ie=UTF8&th=1

43 https://www.thegoodtrade.com/features/natural-aluminum-free-deodorants

44 https://www.revitin.com/.

Glycerin-based soaps are good. [45]

Do not use soap on your body every day. Skin bacteria form a skin microbiome which has many health benefits. Daily water showers work well. Soap may be used for limited areas.

Many sunscreens are not healthy. Avoid those with oxybenzone because, like BPA, is an endocrine disrupter. Avoid sunscreens with vitamin A (or retinol, retinol palmitate). An SPF of 50 or lower is preferable. Non-harmful sunscreen ingredients include titanium dioxide and zinc oxide but avoid nano-sized zinc oxide. Other sunscreen ingredients are neurotoxic (e.g., oxybenzone).

For a review of healthy personal hygiene products, including sunscreens, you are encouraged to visit www.ewg.org

5.6. DETOXIFY REGULARLY.

Planet Earth is extremely polluted with all kind of man-made chemicals, a problem that started with the industrial revolution. Some of these chemicals are causing new genetic defects and are contributors to many medical conditions. It is not possible to be toxin-free any longer. Eating organic food and minimizing exposure to harmful chemicals helps but is not enough. Thus, routine detoxification is recommended.

If you already have any heavy metal poisoning symptoms, you should seek expert medical care. If you do not have any symptoms, you could do a home hair tissue mineral analysis to rule out major toxicities. [46]

SAUNAS. Saunas are well known for their detoxification properties. Toxins accumulate in the fatty (adipose) tissue and are excreted through the skin when sweating. Despite a general aversion to sweating, it is healthy. Infrared saunas are better for detoxification that the old high temperature saunas because the infrared energy penetrates deeper into the fatty tissue. Studies have found larger amount of secreted toxins in the sweat when an infrared sauna is used compare to a conventional sauna. A person in an infrared sauna will sweat at a lower temperature compared to a traditional sauna. A temperature of 125 to 150 degrees Fahrenheit in an infrared sauna is enough. In addition, infrared saunas are more affordable and use less electricity although they take longer to reach the desire temperature.

---

45 https://www.amazon.com/gp/product/B005FAE3UI/ref=ppxyodtbsearchasint itle?ie=UTF8&th=1.

46 https://www.amazon.com/gp/product/B01J6RZTLC/ref=ppx_yo_dt_b_search_asin_title? ie=UTF8&psc=1

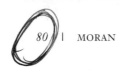

Portable infrared saunas are available as well. [47]

Many gyms have infrared saunas. For home use, a 1- or 2-person sauna is ideal because it plugs directly to an electrical outlet (120 volts in the USA) without the need for specialized wiring. (Regular saunas need 240 volts.) [48] This type of sauna usually comes with speakers for a more enjoyable experience.

SAUNA DETOXIFICATION PROTOCOL. Take immediate release niacin (vitamin B3), which is available over the counter. Do not take the no-flush niacin. Start with 100 mg but this dose may be increased up to 500 mg. After taking niacin, start physical exercise. HIIT (high intensity interval training) is ideal if no contraindications exist and can be done for 16 to 25 minutes. Then get in the sauna. How long? Well, get out if you start feeling uncomfortable. Generally, 20 to 45 minutes is a good guess. You could weigh yourself before and after the sauna. Shower right after using the sauna to wash off all toxins from your skin. Expect to lose 0.4 to 1.2 pounds depending on how long you stay in the sauna, thus rehydrate with water and electrolytes. Initially a large amount of salt is lost in the sweat but with the chronic use of a sauna the salt losses will decrease. Alcohol is contraindicated during or before using a sauna. How often a sauna protocol should be done is quite variable. A healthy person without any symptoms could do it once a week. Somebody with symptoms will require a much more frequent protocol, sometimes daily, to be decided by a medical expert, regarding both frequency and duration.

ANNUAL GENERAL DETOXIFICATION PROTOCOL. This is to detoxify from pesticides and metals. It is meant for asymptomatic patients, to be done for a few weeks once yearly. If you already have symptoms, seek expert medical care. To follow is a combination protocol:

1   Deep purple from BioPure, one scoop daily. It helps to detoxify glyphosate.
2   Rose Hip from BioPure, one scoop twice daily. It helps to detoxify glyphosate.

---

47 https://www.amazon.com/Radiant-Saunas-Rejuvinator-Portable-Personal/dp/B00MX19M9E/ref=sr 1 4?crid=18857XRXEKL37&keywords=portable+infrared+sauna&qid=1557106721&s=lawn-garden&sprefix=portable+infrared+saun%2Clawngarden%2C156&sr=1-4

48 https://www.amazon.com/gp/product/B00A2F99F0/ref=ppx yo dt b search asin title?ie=UTF8&psc=1

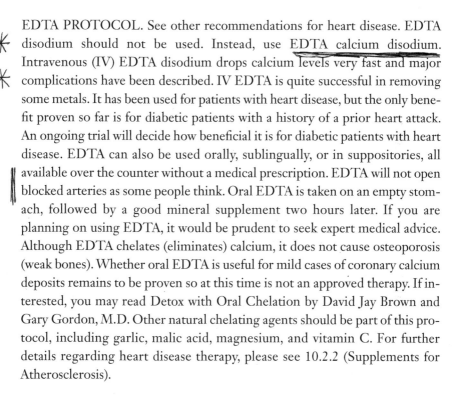

(3) Cilantro herbal tincture, 20 drops daily, to detoxify aluminum. BioPure has one available. Citric acid also eliminates aluminum but not as well as cilantro.

4 Matrix mineral from BioPure or Miracle Minerals from Mimi's. Also helps with glyphosate.

(5) Horsetail tea daily to detoxify aluminum. Synthetic silica will not be effective. For silica to work it must contain small silica particles.

EDTA PROTOCOL. See other recommendations for heart disease. EDTA disodium should not be used. Instead, use EDTA calcium disodium. Intravenous (IV) EDTA disodium drops calcium levels very fast and major complications have been described. IV EDTA is quite successful in removing some metals. It has been used for patients with heart disease, but the only benefit proven so far is for diabetic patients with a history of a prior heart attack. An ongoing trial will decide how beneficial it is for diabetic patients with heart disease. EDTA can also be used orally, sublingually, or in suppositories, all available over the counter without a medical prescription. EDTA will not open blocked arteries as some people think. Oral EDTA is taken on an empty stomach, followed by a good mineral supplement two hours later. If you are planning on using EDTA, it would be prudent to seek expert medical advice. Although EDTA chelates (eliminates) calcium, it does not cause osteoporosis (weak bones). Whether oral EDTA is useful for mild cases of coronary calcium deposits remains to be proven so at this time is not an approved therapy. If interested, you may read Detox with Oral Chelation by David Jay Brown and Gary Gordon, M.D. Other natural chelating agents should be part of this protocol, including garlic, malic acid, magnesium, and vitamin C. For further details regarding heart disease therapy, please see 10.2.2 (Supplements for Atherosclerosis).

OTHER DETOXIFYING PRODUCTS.

- Selenium 100 to 200 mcg daily helps detoxify mercury.
- MSM (methylsulfonylmethane) is essential for detoxification. May take 1,000 to 3,000 mg daily in divided doses. It is more beneficial when taken with vitamin C.
- Soluble fiber like psyllium and vegetables in general.
- Garlic 1 to 4 cloves (crushed) taken daily.
- Vitamin C 2 to 3 grams daily, in divided doses.

6. CANCER PREVENTION AND CANCER RECURRENCE PREVENTION.

VERY IMPORTANT. As it happens with heart disease, most cancers are preventable by understanding epigenetics. Avoid carcinogenics (products that increase cancer risk), eat a healthy diet, control stress, take good care of your microbiome, and take the appropriate supplements. You should increase your body's pH. Many vegetables increase the pH and, in addition, they have many anticancer compounds.

AVOID A HIGH PROTEIN DIET (IMPORTANT).

Typically, a high protein diet is mostly based on animal products. It would be very difficult to eat too much protein on a vegan diet. Protein stimulates the mTOR genetic pathway, as discovered by Dr. Valter Longo, which allows for rapid body growth and stronger muscles. Unfortunately, later in life it is a strong stimulator of cancer growth. Also, a high animal protein diet increases acidity which is rather unhealthy and also increases osteoporosis.

SODIUM BICARBONATE (VERY IMPORTANT).

It is also known as baking soda. Do not confuse with baking powder. Most cancers need an acidic environment to grow. Once the cancer is large enough, it will create its own acidity and bicarbonate will not work any longer, it cannot penetrate and neutralize the cancer produced lactic acidosis. Thus, sodium bicarbonate should be mostly used for PREVENTION. Do not wait until a cancer is well established and diagnosed. One ongoing national trial is testing the role of a much larger bicarbonate dose for cancer therapy but I doubt this approach will be very successful. [49]

For cancer therapy the dose is quite large. For example, a study from the University of Arizona uses 0.5 g/Kg/day. [50]

Some cancers, like melanomas, are not pH dependent and bicarbonate will not help.

For cancer prevention, take one teaspoon (5 grams) of sodium bicarbonate diluted in water twice daily. Or you may add 10 grams to your daily water allowance and drink it throughout the day. Some people purchase water alkalizing

---

49 https://www.ncbi.nlm.nih.gov/pmc/articles/PMC5954837/ *Will cancer cells be defeated by sodium bicarbonate?* Hongtao Zhang* Sci China Life Sci. 2017 Mar; 60(3): 326–328.

50 https://clinicaltrials.gov/ct2/show/NCT02531919

appliances but they are expensive and I am not aware of any specific scientific studies comparing them to oral bicarbonate. To neutralize the bad taste, you may add a small amount of lemon juice or organic apple cider vinegar. Another option is to mix sodium bicarbonate with 10 to 30 ml of apple cider vinegar to eliminate the gas and decrease the need for burping. Then add water before drinking the mixture. You may also add liquid stevia or monk fruit.

Sodium bicarbonate in powder form is very inexpensive. Buy the aluminum free option. You may buy it in tablet form but it is more expensive. Tablets are a good alternative if you are in a hurry or do not want to drink extra fluids.

Hypertension is not a contraindication to using sodium bicarbonate. Contrary to what many people believe, sodium bicarbonate does not increase blood pressure because it does not have any chloride. Table salt (sodium chloride) can increase blood pressure but sodium bicarbonate does not.

I would avoid sodium bicarbonate in patients with congestive heart failure since sodium may retain extra water. In this case, drink apple cider vinegar instead.

Another alternative, if you want to decrease your total sodium intake, is to substitute some of the sodium bicarbonate for potassium bicarbonate. It is also available in powder form. It is contraindicated in patients with kidney failure. You may buy potassium bicarbonate at www.nuts.com

ORGANIC APPLE CIDER VINEGAR.

For those who cannot take bicarbonate or just plainly refuse, you may take 15 ml of organic apple cider vinegar diluted in water twice daily. I favor sodium bicarbonate, although you may take both. Although apple cider vinegar is acidic, once it is metabolized in the body it actually increases (not decreases) the body's pH. You can confirm this fact by testing your urine pH before and after drinking apple cider vinegar.

By increasing the body's pH, like bicarbonate or many vegetables do, it also helps prevent and combat viral infections. This is one of the reasons why a home remedy for cold viral infections mixes 30 ml of apple cider vinegar with 60 ml of water and a good amount of honey. Of course, high quality not adulterated honey also has antiviral and antibacterial properties.

ORGANIC BITTER APRICOT SEEDS.

Apricot seeds contain amygdalin (vitamin B 17), also called laetrile, which is converted into cyanide. This sounds concerning but normal cells have an enzyme capable of neutralizing small amounts of cyanide, something well know by lay people a hundred of years ago. Cancer cells lack this enzyme and should perish.

Nevertheless, at this time vitamin B17 is not used therapeutically because more research is needed. [51]

For prevention (not treatment), 5 to 10 bitter apricot seeds per day may or should decrease the risk of cancer due to their vitamin B 17 content (see *World without Cancer. The Story of Vitamin B17* by G. Edward Griffin). Avoid eating a large number of apricot seeds in the beginning. Some people have been successful increasing the number of ingested apricot seeds over time but they usually do it because they already have a cancer. Laetrile is not FDA approved for cancer therapy in the USA, thus no medication is available. In my opinion, bitter apricot seeds should be used in a comprehensive protocol to prevent cancer from happening in the first place.

Do not buy the non-bitter apricot seeds. If they are not bitter is because they do not have amygdalin and will not have any beneficial effect against cancer.

Another alternative, if you can find them, is bitter almonds. Maybe they are available in other countries but they are not commercially available in USA. If everything fails, remember, amygdalin is found in apple seeds also, and so you may eat the seeds of one apple once a day.

BRASSICA TEA OR COFFEE.

Brassica tea or coffee comes with truebloc, a patented substance from broccoli that has good anti-cancer properties. For cancer prevention, drink one cup of tea or coffee daily. To decrease the risk of a cancer recurrence, drink at least two cups daily.

VITAMIN D3 SUPPLEMENTS.

In a scientific study, Dr. McDonell noticed women with a vitamin D level greater than 60 ng/ml had an 80 percent decreased risk of suffering breast cancer compared to women whose vitamin D level was less than 20 ng/ml. Vitamin D3 is a critical hormone-like product needed for many functions, including the immune system. For this purpose, a much higher intake is needed than just for calcium absorption and bone health.

Vitamin D supplements—4,000 to 5,000 IU—if you do not get enough sun exposure should reduce cancer risk also because it is a powerful stimulator of

51 https://www.ncbi.nlm.nih.gov/pmc/articles/PMC5986699/ Effects of the Gut microbiota on Amygdalin and its use as an anti-cancer therapy: Substantial review on the key components involved in altering dose efficacy and toxicity. Vani Jaswal et al. Biochem Biophys Rep. 2018 Jul; 14: 125–132.

the immune system. Higher doses might be needed for other indications but anything higher than 10,000 IU daily requires monitoring blood testing to rule out toxic levels of vitamin D.

✷ AVOID CARCINOGENS OR CARCINOGEN-LIKE SUBSTANCES OR PRODUCTS.

Avoid hormonal disrupting chemicals, like plastic with BPA or phthalates. This is another good reason to avoid plastics for any type of food storage.

TO FOLLOW IS A NON-COPYRIGHTED LIST OF RECOMMENDATIONS FROM AN INTERNET BLOG REGARDING CANCER OR RECURRENT CANCER PREVENTION. I ADDED THE LINKS. YOU CAN DRAW YOUR OWN CONCLUSIONS.

Most cancers are caused by:
- Acidic Body Environment
- Intoxication with heavy metals and similar substances like Flouride, Aluminum, Mercury, Lead...
- Strong hormone imbalance endocrine disrupting chemical, xenoestrogens and so on (BPA is one of the most common ones)

Things you have to avoid:
- All cosmetic products that contain aluminum and if possible all of the "common known" cosmetic products like soap, shower gel, cremes, shampoos...
- Avoid anything where food comes into contact with aluminum like aluminum pans, aluminum foil or other types of aluminum containers and packaging

WHY YOU SHOULD USE ALUMINUM-FREE DEODORANT
https://www.globalhealingcenter.com/natural-health/why-you-should-use-aluminum-free-deodorant/

NEW RESEARCH INDICATES ALUMINUM IN DEODORANT LINKED TO BREAST CANCER
https://www.globalhealingcenter.com/natural-health/aluminum-and-breast-cancer/

NEW STUDY LINKS ALUMINUM TO OSTEOPOROSIS AND ALZHEIMER'S DISEASE

https://www.globalhealingcenter.com/natural-health/new-study-links-aluminum-to-osteoporosis-and-alzheimers-disease/

- Completely avoid trans fats

HOW PARTIALLY-HYDROGENATED OILS AND TRANS FATS DESTROY YOUR HEALTH

https://www.naturalnews.com/027445fatfatstrans.html

TRANS FATS INCREASE RISK OF DEATH BY MORE THAN A THIRD, STUDY FINDS

https://www.naturalnews.com/051079transfatsheartattackhydro-genatedoils.h tml

TRANS FATS IN JUNK FOOD IMPAIR BRAIN FUNCTION, CAUSE MEMORY LOSS

https://www.naturalnews.com/050182transfatsmemoryjunkfood.html

- Avoid foods with preservatives like sodium nitrite [NaNO2] [E-250] and also foods containing glutamate (E6XX), especially MSG (Monosodium Glutamate E621)

THE HARMFUL EFFECTS OF MONOSODIUM GLUTAMATE (MSG)

https://www.globalhealingcenter.com/natural-health/harmful-effects-of-monosodium-glutamate-msg/

MONOSODIUM GLUTAMATE AND ALL ITS HIDDEN FORMS: YEAST EXTRACT, TVP, HYDROLYZED PROTEINS AND MORE

https://www.naturalnews.com/045741monosodiumglutamateyeastextracthydr olyzedproteins.html

MONOSODIUM GLUTAMATE (MSG): IS THIS SILENT KILLER HIDING IN YOUR FOOD

https://www.naturalnewsblogs.com/monosodium-glutamate-msg-silent-killer-hiding-food/

- Avoid carbohydrates and especially sugar as much as possible because consuming them is like "feeding" your cancer cells

WHY IS REFINED SUGAR SO BAD FOR YOUR HEALTH?
https://www.globalhealingcenter.com/natural-health/health-concerns-of-refined-sugar/

SUGAR AND CANCER
https://www.globalhealingcenter.com/newsletter/2004/february/articles.php?id=1

THE HIDDEN TRUTH ABOUT ENRICHED WHITE FLOUR
https://www.globalhealingcenter.com/natural-health/enriched-white-flour/

- Avoid artificial sweeteners also because they are at least as harmful as sugar if not more harmful like in the case of aspartame

THE HEALTH DANGERS OF ASPARTAME
https://www.globalhealingcenter.com/natural-health/health-dangers-of-aspartame/

THE TWO MOST DANGEROUS ARTIFICIAL SWEETENERS
https://www.globalhealingcenter.com/natural-health/two-of-the-most-dangerous-artificial-sweeteners/

 Avoid BPA especially if your cancer is in your genital areas (prostate, breast, ovaries). Many foods and beverages these days are packaged in plastic containers that contain BPA or containers (like plastic bottles) that are laced with BPA (like cans).

6 REASONS BPA IS A TOXIC POISON
https://www.globalhealingcenter.com/natural-health/6-reasons-bpa/

NEW STUDY PROVES ANY AMOUNT OF BPA HARMS REPRODUCTIVE HEALTH
https://www.globalhealingcenter.com/natural-health/new-study-proves-bpa-harms-reproductive-health/

10 THINGS TO KNOW ABOUT BPA

https://www.globalhealingcenter.com/natural-health/10-things-to-know-about-bpa/

BPA-FREE DOES NOT MEAN SAFE

https://www.globalhealingcenter.com/natural-health/bpa-free-does-not-mean-safe/

STUDY: BPA DISRUPTS PROSTATE HEALTH

https://www.globalhealingcenter.com/natural-health/study-bpa-disrupts-prostate-health/

Avoid fluoride especially in toothpaste and drinking water! Processed foods you buy might also have been made with fluoridated water.

FLUORIDE: DAILY EXPOSURE TO POISON

https://www.globalhealingcenter.com/natural-health/fluoride-poison-on-tap-documentary/

THE DANGERS OF FLUORIDE

https://www.globalhealingcenter.com/natural-health/how-safe-is-fluoride/

WHY YOU SHOULD REDUCE YOUR EXPOSURE TO FLUORIDE

https://www.globalhealingcenter.com/natural-health/reduce-your-exposure-to-fluoride/

DETOXIFY AND HEAL YOUR BODY

Take 1 or better 2 teaspoons of pure baking soda (sodium bicarbonate or sodium hydrogen carbonate) every day before you go to sleep. This is one of the most important steps to curing cancer!!! Baking soda or the sodium to be exact is THE natural ph level regulator of the body so as long as there is enough sodium available the body can neutralize most harmful substances (acids) easily. If for whatever reason you also need to take baking soda during the day then you should mix the baking soda with fresh pressed lemon juice to avoid getting diarrhea.

BAKING SODA AND LEMON? POWERFUL HEALING COMBINATION FOR CANCER

https://www.naturalnewsblogs.com/baking-soda-lemon-powerful-healing-combination-cancer/

BAKING SODA, CANCER AND FUNGUS

https://www.naturalnews.com/035876bakingsodacancer fungus.html

Switch to organic food

EFFECTS OF PESTICIDES

https://www.globalhealingcenter.com/natural-health/effects-of-pesticides/

Completely switch to natural derived cosmetic products. Baking soda-based deodorants are very effective and healthy!

4 WAYS TO MAKE YOUR OWN ALL-NATURAL DEODORANT

https://www.liveabout.com/diy-all-natural-deodorant-1387817

SOME COMPANIES THAT OFFER GOOD NATURAL COSMETIC PRODUCT:

Eco Cosmetics https://eco-naturkosmetik.de/?lang=en

Weleda https://www.weleda.com/

Lavera https://www.lavera.de/en/

Just check at what shops you can buy their products

Eat lots of healthy fats like coconut oil and hemp oil. I suggest to switch from all fat you use for cooking to coconut oil and additionally take 1 Tablespoon of organic, native, cold-pressed hemp oil every day! Forget the mainstream narrative about fats, as good fats are absolutely essential to health and the good fats do not make you fat! Forget calorie counting as proteins and good fats are not going to be burned but instead be used to repair and rebuild the cells of your body. The only thing that is good for nothing but calories are carbohydrates.

WHAT ARE FATS? ARE ALL DIETARY FATS BAD?

https://www.globalhealingcenter.com/natural-health/what-are-fats/

THE HEALTH BENEFITS OF OMEGA 3, 6, 9 FATTY ACIDS AND EPA & DHA

https://www.globalhealingcenter.com/natural-health/benefits-of-omega-3-6-9-fatty-acids/

Stop using regular table salt and switch to Himalayan crystal salt

THE BENEFITS OF HIMALAYAN SALT

https://www.globalhealingcenter.com/natural-health/himalayan-crystal-salt-benefits/

THE HEALTH DANGERS OF TABLE SALT

https://www.globalhealingcenter.com/natural-health/dangers-of-salt/

Supplement your nutrition with Chlorella and Spirulina. My suggestion is to take 10 "tablets" of each in the morning and evening

CHLORELLA PREMIUM SUPERFOOD DELIVERS POTENT NUTRITION, DETOXIFICATION

https://www.naturalnews.com/030030chlorellasuperfood.html

SPIRULINA SHOWN TO PREVENT AND TREAT CANCERS WHILE BOOSTING IMMUNE SYSTEM FUNCTION

https://www.naturalnews.com/008421.html

SPIRULINA: A BUDGET FRIENDLY SUPER FOOD AND ANSWER TO FOOD SCARCITY

https://www.naturalnews.com/023337.html

Supplement Iodine: While Himalayan crystal salt and chlorella already contain some good iodine, it might still be a good idea to additionally supplement with monoatomic (nascent, unbound) iodine to get a good deal of toxins out of your body fast.

WHAT IS IODINE?
https://www.globalhealingcenter.com/natural-health/what-is-iodine/

SURVIVAL SHIELD X-2 - NASCENT IODINE
http://www.infowarsshop.com/

DETOXADINE
https://www.globalhealingcenter.com/nascent-iodine-detoxadine.html

Get the aluminum out of your body! One of the best ways to remove aluminum is silica-based supplements like "horsetail"

WHAT IS HORSETAIL? DISCOVER ITS BENEFITS AND USES
https://www.globalhealingcenter.com/natural-health/what-is-horsetail/

5 BENEFITS OF DIATOMACEOUS EARTH
https://www.globalhealingcenter.com/natural-health/5-benefits-of-diatomaceous-earth/

WHAT IS SILICA AND HOW CAN IT SUPPORT YOUR HEALTH?
https://www.globalhealingcenter.com/natural-health/what-is-silica-support-health/

4 WAYS TO DETOXIFY ALUMINUM FROM YOUR LIFE
https://www.globalhealingcenter.com/natural-health/detoxify-aluminum/

CHOOSING THE RIGHT COOKWARE
https://www.globalhealingcenter.com/natural-health/choosing-the-right-cookware/

- Replace Sugar and Artificial sweeteners with stevia and xylitol Make sure the xylitol has been derived from organic sources!

7 REASONS WHY STEVIA IS BETTER THAN REFINED SUGAR
https://www.globalhealingcenter.com/natural-health/stevia/

DISCOVER THE BENEFITS OF XYLITOL, THE SAFE ALTERNATIVE TO SUGAR
https://www.naturalnews.com/042855xylitolsafealternativessugar-substitute.ht ml

- Take high dosages of good antioxidants Vitamin C (at least 1,000 to 2,000mg each day and spread out during the day 2 to 3 times, additionally Vitamin E) and if it is not in oil form make sure you take some oil/fat with it. Maybe combine it with the hemp oil.
 Grape Seed Extract (OPC) is a very powerful antioxidant that boosts the effect of vitamin C/E, natural blood thinner, helps with detox , fights cancer cells and more...

VITAMIN C SHOWN TO ANNIHILATE CANCER
https://www.naturalnews.com/049957_vitamin_c_cancer_natural_remedies.html

16 FOODS HIGH IN VITAMIN C
https://www.globalhealingcenter.com/natural-health/foods-high-in-vitamin-c/

WHY IS VITAMIN E IMPORTANT TO YOUR HEALTH?
https://www.globalhealingcenter.com/natural-health/vitamin-e-health-benefits/

VITAMIN E KILLS OFF CANCER CELLS AND PREVENTS THEIR REPRODUCTION, STUDY FINDS
https://www.naturalnews.com/050646vitaminEcancerstudydisease prevention.html

HEALTH BENEFITS OF GRAPE SEED EXTRACT
https://www.naturalnews.com/042417grapeseedextracthealthbene-fitsantioxidants.html

GRAPE SEED EXTRACT MORE EFFECTIVE THAN CHEMOTHERAPY IN ADVANCED CANCER

https://www.naturalnews.com/050231grapeseedextractchemotherapycancertreatments.html

GRAPE SEED EXTRACT KILLS LEUKEMIA CELLS IN LABORATORY

https://www.naturalnews.com/025521grapeseedextractleukemia-cancer.html

- High Dosage Vitamin D3
  I personally take 20,000 IU Vitamin D every day so I suggest you take at least that much as well. If it is not in oil form already, combine it with the taking of the hemp oil.

VITAMIN D HALTS GROWTH OF BREAST CANCER TUMORS
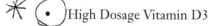

https://www.naturalnews.com/025495VitaminDbreastcancer.html

- Take hormone balancing supplements.

WEBINAR: NATURAL SOLUTIONS FOR HORMONAL IMBALANCE

https://www.globalhealingcenter.com/natural-health/hormonal-imbalance/

STINGING NETTLE FOR PROSTATE HEALTH

https://www.globalhealingcenter.com/natural-health/stinging-nettle-prostate-health/

CHRYSIN IS NATURAL ALTERNATIVE TO TOXIC BREAST CANCER DRUGS

https://www.naturalnews.com/026086cancerdrugchrysin.html

- Eat apricot seeds every day. They contain "Vitamin B17" that kills off cancer cells while not harming healthy cells.

APRICOT SEEDS KILL CANCER CELLS WITHOUT SIDE EFFECTS
https://www.naturalnews.com/027088cancerlaetrilecure.html

HOW LAETRILE OR B17 FROM APRICOT SEEDS KILLS
https://www.naturalnews.com/031336laetrilecancercells.html

- Clean your gut and rebuild a healthy gut flora.

5 Benefits of Colon Cleansing
https://www.globalhealingcenter.com/natural-health/5-benefits-of-colon-cleansing/

CLEANSING INSTRUCTIONS FOR DR. GROUPS 7-DAY OXYGEN COLON CLEANSE:
https://www.oxypowder.com/instructions/

3 REASONS HEALTHY GUT FLORA IS IMPORTANT
https://www.globalhealingcenter.com/natural-health/3-reasons-healthy-gut-flora-are-important/

7. OTHER RECOMMENDATIONS

7.1. MICROWAVE OVENS

Avoid cooking meals in microwave ovens because the food will lose nutritional value. It seems reasonable to use microwaves ovens occasionally to reheat meals. This will not produce any toxic products like what happens when food is overheated on the stove or in a traditional oven. Thus, it is better to reheat food in the microwave then with other means that might overheat the food and change the quality of its fat content.

7.2. GROUNDING (EARTHING).

Earthing happens when the body, which as a positive electric charge, touches the earth, which has a negative charge, like walking barefoot on the beach. When this happens, electrons from the earth enter the body. These electrons work as free radical scavengers decreasing inflammation in general, and having many other beneficial health effects. Earthing is also called grounding.

Do daily earthing or grounding—may do with commercially available devices—whenever you can. Even limited time will be beneficial although longer times are more effective.

Best earthing is walking barefoot on the beach exposed to sunlight. Unfortunately this is often not possible for those living in the northern states. A reasonable alternative is to place a copper rod in the ground by your house, then bring a wire into your home. Although grounding can be done using grounded electrical outlets, this is thought by some to be a poor idea do to the negative effects of the "dirty alternating electrical current."

For scientific literature supporting earthing see "OTHER REFERENCES" at the end.

7.3. CIRCADIAN RHYTHM (IMPORTANT).

Sleep about 8 hours a day, always going to bed at about the same time. Some people might need only 7 hours. All body cells have a circadian rhythm. Avoid blue light at night. Blue light, like LED light and electronic devices screens (e.g., computers, cellular phones, TV screens, etc.) interfere with the secretion of melatonin at night. Melatonin is the sleep hormone, needed for a good night rest. It is also a powerful antioxidant.

It is healthier when people go to bed before midnight, ideally at about the same time. People working the night shift lose life expectancy. Even worse is when employees are required to work different shifts, which has serious long-term health consequences.

Many major world accidents have occurred during the night shift. In some countries working more than 24 hours is illegal, although this probably to protect the public.

7.4. LED LIGHTS

LED lights save energy but may cause retinal damage by increasing the risk of macular degeneration and blindness. To this respect, the French government already had issued a warning many years ago. A study from Madrid, Spain, also showed retinal damage with exposure to LED light.

LED lights are very disruptive. They interfere with normal circadian rhythm if used at night because of their blue light spectrum. The body is cheated into thinking it is still day time and will not produce melatonin well. Melatonin is needed for a good sleep cycle. Thus, avoid screens (laptop and desktop computers, TVs, etc.) unless protective glasses are worn. Another option is to have a software changing the type of light emitted by the screen, like f.lux (may download at https://justgetflux.com/).

Avoid LEDs at night a few hours before bedtime, or at least dim the lights. I changed back to incandescent lights in the living room and kitchen.

7.5. DONATE BLOOD IF ABLE.

Donate blood at least once a year. It decreases the risk of heart disease. If you do not have anemia, donating blood twice annually is a good idea. Also check your blood ferritin level. High ferritin levels correlate with heart disease and colon cancer. Although hemoglobin needs iron, too much iron is very toxic.

If your blood cannot be used for a transfusion, you can still request a phlebotomy (blood is removed and discarded).

See "OTHER REFERENCES" at the end.

7.6. AMALGAMS WITH MERCURY

This issue is very controversial. I would leave the amalgams alone (do not remove them) if you do not have any mercury poisoning symptoms and your hair tissue mineral analysis does not show any toxic levels. Removal of amalgams that have mercury carries a significant risk of mercury poisoning. If you decide to replace your mercury amalgams, go to a dentist who has the appropriate suctioning equipment and expertise.

7.7. VACCINES IN GENERAL.

Do your own research since this has become a political issue with big corporate financial interests at stake. Thus, I will mostly avoid this topic but plenty of information is available in books and online.

Combination of vaccines and glyphosate. The combination of (a) aluminum, mercury, or vaccines that have aluminum (or mercury but this is quite unusual now) and (b) glyphosate (= Round Up®, which is present in GMO foods and some non-GMO foods) causes autism, dementia, and many other problem based on MIT senior researcher Dr. Stephanie Seneff. Her scientific articles are available at the MIT webpage. In addition, two studies have shown the flu vaccine negatively affects the immune system. Too much of a good thing might be harmful. Developed countries with most vaccinations have the highest infant mortality [52]; increasing numbers of vaccine doses correlate

---

52 http://www.ncbi.nlm.nih.gov/pmc/articles/PMC3170075/

with infant hospitalizations and deaths [53]. Concerns exist about increased vaccination causing metabolic syndrome. [54]

Glyphosate has also been found to correlate with many other conditions, including some cancers, inflammatory bowel disease, etc. In addition, glyphosate correlates with many other mental conditions, like ADD (attention deficit disorder), depression, etc.

In USA patients cannot sue for any related vaccine complications (exception is for a vaccine that cannot be used for children like the shingles vaccine). This is based on a federal statute which has been upheld constitutional by the United States Supreme Court. The harmed individual can seek financial compensation from a Federal fund, the National Vaccine Injury Compensation Program. [55] Although vaccines are considered safe, this program has already paid out more than three billion dollars. Some lawyers have stated not to try to file a claim on your own as the likelihood of getting a monetary award would be slim or none. Thus, an expert attorney in this field must be hired.

7.8. INLUENZA VACCINE.

The influenza vaccine (flu shot) is somewhat effective in preventing influenza (the flu). Based on several years reported by the CDC (Center for Disease Control and Prevention), average effectiveness for the fourteen years from 2004/05 to 2017/18 was close to 41 percent. [56] Independent researchers tend to give slightly lower effectiveness numbers. The flu shot carries a very small but significant risk of developing a major neurological disease called Guillain-Barré syndrome.

Most compensable vaccine related injuries are paid for complications from the flu shot (2,949 out of 4,311, thus 68.4 percent). [57]

Thus, you should carefully balance the risks and benefits of the flu shot (influenza vaccine). In many studies, effectiveness has not been found in patients 65 or older. In addition, the very young get less protection from the flu shot.

---

53 http://www.ncbi.nlm.nih.gov/pubmed/22531966

54 https://acenewsdesk.wordpress.com/2014/11/11/study-review-of-vaccine-induced-immune-overload-resulting-epidemics-of-type-1-diabetes-metabolic-syndrome/

55 https://www.hrsa.gov/vaccine-compensation/index.html

56 See https://www.cdc.gov/flu/vaccines-work/effectiveness-studies.htm (accessed May 27, 2019).

57 https://www.hrsa.gov/vaccine-compensation/index.html (accessed May 27, 2019).

7.9 AUTISM.

Stay away from the combination of aluminum-glyphosate because it seems to be the main cause of autism. This combination also contributes to dementia. Thus, do not eat any GMO food. Do not get any shots or vaccines that have aluminum (or mercury). Do not expose your body to any aluminum, no exceptions.

7.10 SUNLIGHT & EXPOSURE.

Sunlight has many health benefits, some probably still unknown. Like with anything else, moderation is the key. Excessive sunlight is the main cause of skin cancers, as well as wrinkles. Exposure of a large percentage of the body to sunlight for 15 to 20 minutes per day is enough. This will produce several thousand units of vitamin D, which is never toxic when obtained this natural way. Sunlight helps the immune system and decrease cancer risk. It also decreases depression.

7.11. BROWN FAT.

Increasing the amount of the body's brown fat amount is healthy although from a practical point of view it might be difficult to achieve. Brown fat is metabolically active, thus it uses energy instead of storing it, warming up your body. Brown fat explains why people can get used to working in cold conditions. Cold showers, cold baths, significant cooler bedroom at night are ways to increase brown fat. Thus, it keeps you warm and also helps with weight loss. A simple way to increase brown fat is 2- to 4-minute cold showers daily. The Wim Hof method combines cold showers with breathing exercises, not just to increase brown fat but also to control stress and improve the immune system. [58]

It is more difficult to have brown fat in tropical zones, thus those people should be encouraged to exercise more to compensate for the lack or lesser amount of brown fat.

8. RECOMMENDATIONS FOR AUTOIMMUNE DISEASES

No magic cure for autoimmune diseases exists. The incidence of many autoimmune diseases, like multiple sclerosis and rheumatoid arthritis, has increased over the last few decades. Women are more prone than men. Often patients have low vitamin D blood levels. Although the underlying genetic predisposition cannot be cured, the triggering mechanisms can be discontinued.

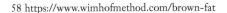

58 https://www.wimhofmethod.com/brown-fat

Several authors have published books with good advice on how to improve autoimmune diseases. *The Wahls Protocol* by Terry Wahls, MD. *Put Your Heart in Your Mouth* by Dr. Natascha Campbell-McBride, MD, and *The Autoimmune Fix* by Tom O'Bryan, DC, CCN, DACBN.

RECCOMENDATIONS:

- Eat a ketogenic organic diet, as recommended by Dr. Steven Gundry in his book *The Plant Paradox*. Thus, avoid lectins, gluten, grains, and dairy products. Again, all food must be organic.
- Avoid processed foods and eating out at restaurants.
- Cook at low temperatures (less than 212 degrees Fahrenheit).
- The omega 6 to 3 fatty acids ratio should be one to one (no more than 3:1).
- Do not eat more than 20 g/day of saturated fats.
- Take a daily probiotic supplement or eat probiotic foods, like sauerkraut.
- Eat daily prebiotics, like inulin, onions, etc.
- Water should be filtered, ideally by reverse osmosis. No other drinks except for tea and coffee.
- Avoid harmful products:
- Only use organic sunscreen or cosmetic products.
- Use organic detergent.
- Glycerin based soap for hand and/or body washing.
- Do not use any bed sheets that have been treated with fire retardant chemicals.
- Use a healthy tooth paste without fluoride, like Revitin, which is a prebiotic.
- Avoid antiperspirant deodorants. Make sure deodorants are aluminum free.
- Skip taking a bath or a shower for a couple of weeks to allow the skin microbiome to recover. Then shower daily but mostly with water, without soap or soap for few areas.
- Do not use any plastic containers to store food.
- Cook with stainless steel or ceramic.
- Avoid unnecessary vaccines.
- Avoid broad spectrum antibiotics if possible.
- Clean your home air with a HEPA filter air purifier.

- Consult with a functional medicine physician to rule out heavy metal intoxication or mineral imbalances, as well as for appropriate therapy. A screening hair tissue mineral analysis is a good idea.
- What to do with mercury amalgams is controversial.
- Detoxify your body. Several protocols are available.
- Low dose naltrexone has been used with good results. It will need a prescription and medical supervision. Starting dose is one mg/day, increasing up to 4 to 5 mg/day. It is taken at night. A contraindication is the current use of narcotics. See *The LDN Book* by Linda Elsegood.

SUPPLEMENTS:

- Vitamin D3 starting at 5,000 to 10,000 IU daily. Check blood levels to make sure a high level is obtained. May increase dose accordingly. Vitamin D helps immune system regulation.
- Estriol has been used.
- Melatonin in large doses to help regulate the immune system.
- Alpha lipoic acid has been used for multiple sclerosis.
- Glutathione, vitamin C, vitamin E.
- Coenzyme Q 10 in the ubiquinol form.
- Meditation to control stress.

9. PAIN KILLERS.

NSAIDS have many side effects. Avoid them. A short course of ibuprofen is acceptable, e.g., after a surgical procedure. NSAIDS should not be taken on a chronic basis because they can cause bleeding stomach ulcers, colitis, high blood pressure, kidney damage, and disrupt the gut barrier contributing to a "leaky gut" (which causes many health problems, including autoimmune diseases). In addition, with the exception of aspirin, NSAIDS like ibuprofen and naproxen increase the risk of heart disease, heart failure, and stroke. You will be able to see this warning on the bottle, as required by the FDA (Food and Drug Administration).

Acetominophen (Tylenol) is not as dangerous as NSAIDS but has caused acute liver failure (and death) when mixed with alcohol. It may also cause other not-well known problems. Avoid it if you can.

Safer pain killers include Boswellia extract, which is also an anti-inflammatory but does not cause a leaky gut, and white willow bark. Both are over the counter medications.

If you need an anti-inflammatory medication, use turmeric. It is not absorbed well but in a pill form already comes with other products, like BioPerine, to improve absorption. If you take turmeric in a powder form, add a small amount of organic black pepper, it will increase absorption. It might take days or a few weeks for turmeric to work well.

The main way to deal with chronic pain is curing the underlying condition, or even better, prevent the problem from happening (e.g., prevent osteoarthritis by eating healthy, maintaining a normal weight, doing weight-bearing exercises, etc.).

10. SUPPLEMENTS

No supplement can counteract the harmful effects of an unhealthy diet.

10.1. SUPPLEMENTS IN GENERAL.

Supplement recommendations are difficult, controversial to a certain degree, and a moving target. Obviously, not everybody will require the same supplements, which will be based on age, sex, and other personal conditions.

10.1.1. VITAMIN C (IMPORTANT).

The minimal daily requirements of vitamin C are to prevent major deficiencies but are not enough for good bodily function, like growing new cartilage in the joints. Vitamin C is water soluble, thus it does not have to be taken with fat or meals. In fact, because it increases iron absorption it is not a bad idea to take it in between meals. For this reason, patients with some iron accumulation diseases should not take vitamin C supplements unless excess iron is eliminated.

The best vitamin C is the one found in food, like citrus fruits. This is true for all vitamins. The food should be eaten raw because heat will destroy vitamin C. A simple advice is to drink the juice of a lemon or lime daily because it does not have any fructose and it offers other health benefits, in this case increasing the body's pH once it is metabolized.

Liposomal vitamin C is more expensive but a better option. Regular vitamin C supplements are quickly excreted in the urine. The recommended dose is 500 to 1,000 mg twice a day. Higher dose can be taken since it has no major side effects. For somebody with arterial vascular disease (e.g., coronary artery disease) or with osteoarthritis, take 1,000 mg twice daily or even three times daily. This dose is also recommended if you are trying to detoxify your body from heavy metals.

Vitamin C has a short life and ideally should be taken several times daily. A solution to this problem is taking sustained release vitamin C, which will last for 24 hours.

10.1.2. MAGNESIUM (VERY IMPORTANT).

It is estimated that 70 to 80 percent of the world's population has some degree of magnesium deficiency. Soil magnesium has been low or depleted for many decades. A magnesium deficiency can cause many medical problems, including muscle cramps, restless leg syndrome, atrial fibrillation (irregular heart beat) and other arrhythmias, heart attacks (due to increase calcium deposits), hypertension, osteoporosis, failure to respond to calcium supplements after thyroid or parathyroid surgery, irregular heartbeats after open heart surgery, fatigue and muscle weakness, mental disorders, and worsening asthma among others. Dietary calcium will not prevent osteoporosis if a magnesium deficiency is present.

Many types of magnesium are available. AVOID magnesium oxide because it only has an 8 percent absorption rate. Potassium citrate is a reasonable alternative. It is relatively well absorbed and well priced. It can be purchased in powder form to avoid other non-active ingredients. Other forms of magnesium are absorbed better but are more expensive. For example, magnesium orotate, magnesium glycenate, magnesium L-threonate, magnesium gluconate, magnesium chloride, magnesium aspartate, and ionic magnesium.

RDA for magnesium is 310 to 420 mg/day but some experts recommend twice as much, certainly for patients with hypertension.

If you develop loose stools, start with a smaller dose divided and taken a few times daily, then increase the dose slowly. Also, avoid magnesium oxide and take a chelated magnesium.

For a detailed review you may read *The Miracle of Magnesium* by Carolyn Dean and The Magnesium Factor by Mildred Seelig. Or check the magnesium webpage www.mgwater.com

10.1.3. VITAMIN D-3 (VERY IMPORTANT).

If you can expose your body to the sun rays for 15 to 20 minutes daily, no vitamin D3 supplementation is needed. Unfortunately, a large percentage of the population is vitamin D deficient and has a lower level that is not ideal to support normal body functions, like the immune system. The official recommended dose might be enough to support the bones but not for the immune system or other functions. Vitamin D is really not a vitamin, but a hormone-like product that plays a very important role in maintaining good health. Patients with autoimmune diseases often have a low vitamin D level. Vitamin D deficiency increases the risk of coronary artery disease, aortic valve calcifications, cancers, and overall mortality.

Take one pill of 4,000 or 5,000 IU daily, with a meal. Vitamin D is liposoluble, which means it must be taken with fat for good absorption. No toxicity has been reported with doses up to 4,000 IU. As far as I know 5,000 IU, which is a typical pill dose in USA, should be safe for almost everybody. Do not exceed 10,000 IU unless you follow blood levels. Nevertheless, Tiago Henriques recommends starting with 10,000 IU daily (see his book *How Not to Die with True High-Dose Vitamin D Therapy*). If you do this for more than a few months, it would be prudent to check your blood level. Vitamin D toxicity is very rare but it has been reported. Persistent toxic blood levels of vitamin D can lead to complications, like hypercalcemia (high blood calcium level, can cause kidney stones and other problems).

No toxicity occurs from natural vitamin D production, regardless of length of sun exposure. If obtaining your vitamin D from sun exposure, do not take a shower with soap for a few hours or you will wash off the vitamin D. Only half of the pre-vitamin D is absorbed within the first two hours.

People with autoimmune conditions should maximize their blood vitamin levels to the highest safe level because vitamin D is a good immune system regulator. In this case, blood level testing is in order to make sure a high level is obtained.

10.1.4. VITAMIN K2.

A. MK-7 (VERY IMPORTANT).

Vitamin K exists as vitamin K1, used for clotting, and vitamin K2 which is used by the body to form normal bones and avoid calcium deposits in other locations. People in Western societies are usually deficient in vitamin K2. Without enough vitamin K2, calcium is not deposited in the bones but in the wrong places, like the coronary arteries, the aorta, the skin (causing wrinkles), and in the crystalline (causing cataracts). Survival correlates well with amount of calcium deposited in the arteries. Coronary artery disease is usually due to calcification secondary to inflammation and contributing factors are vitamin K2 and magnesium deficiencies. Prevent chronic inflammation and calcification and you will eliminate or greatly reduce heart attacks. Green leafy vegetables have vitamin K1 but not vitamin K2. Vitamin K1 is used by the liver to make clotting factors but K1 does not decrease arterial calcifications. Vitamin K1 deficiency is quite rare.

In Japan, the consumption of vitamin K2 is much higher because many Japanese eat natto, a naturally reach vitamin K2 food. About 3.5 ounces (100 grams) of natto have 1,100 mcg of vitamin K2 MK-7. Be aware that MK-7 is measured in micrograms (mcg) not in milligrams (mg).

Take a supplement of at least 90 to 120 mcg of vitamin K2 daily, always with food because it is liposoluble, in other words it needs fat to be absorbed. Clinical trials are being done with MK-7 not MK-4. The MK-7 subtype is potentially more effective because it lasts longer and it only has to be taken once a day. To follow are dosing guidelines. Infants up to 6 months of age, 2. 0 mcg. Infants 7 to 12 months, 2.5 mcg. Children 1 to 3 years old, 30 mcg. Children 4 to 8 years old, 55 mcg. Children 9 to 13 years old, 60 mcg. Children 14 to 18 years old, 75 mcg. Adults 19 years and older, 90 mcg for women and 120 mcg for men. [59]

MK-7 should be taken in the trans isomer because it is the biologically active one. The cis isomer is not found in nature and is not active or not much. MK-7 produced by organic synthesis is always trans. If produced by fermentation, good extraction and purification techniques are needed to obtain the trans MK-7 exclusively. Some MK-7 from China have been found to only have 15 to 30 percent of trans. You want to buy a supplement with 100 percent trans MK-7.

To prevent osteoporosis some experts think it is better to take a higher dose of MK-7 of 180 mcg daily. Kate Rheaume-Bleue in her book *Vitamin K2 and the Calcium Paradox* recommends taking at least 240 mcg daily for menopausal or post menopausal women, as well as for prediabetics, diabetics, and over-weight people.

If you already have osteoporosis or heart disease (e.g., calcium in the coronary arteries on a CT scan or known arterial heart disease) a higher dose seem to be reasonable. An ongoing trial to stop or reverse coronary artery calcium is using 360 mcg/day. Another ongoing clinical trial to decrease calcium in the aorta is using 720 mcg/day. A third study is using 1,000 mcg but only three times weekly, thus an average of 428 mcg/day. It might take a few years for those results to become available, in the meantime the best dose of vitamin MK-7 to reverse arterial calcium or plaque remains unknown. So far, no side effects from vitamin K2 administration have been reported.

MK-7 at doses of up to 47 mcg/day does not interfere with blood thinners. People on blood thinners should check with their cardiologist or primary care

---

59 Guideline source https://www.canprev.ca/wp-content/themes/Avada-Child-Theme/docs/Vitamin-K2-primer.pdf?pdf=Vitamin-K2-Primer

provider before taking MK-7 supplements. A higher dose will probably interfere with vitamin K antagonists, like coumadin (warfarin). It is not clear to me whether this is applicable to the new oral blood thinner medications, like Pradaxa (dabigatran), Eliquis (apixaban), Xarelto (rivaroxaban) etc. because their mechanism of action is different and vitamin K2 does not increase clotting in a person who is not on blood thinners (anticoagulants). Thus, you should consult with your cardiologist.

Please remember, MK-7 is not a magic fix-all solution, it still needs to be taking in conjunction with a healthy diet (which will provide the calcium), vitamin D3 and magnesium supplements.

Further information can be found at www.vitamink2.org or vitamink2.org

B. MK-4

Vitamin MK-7 is found in fermented food, like natto and some cheeses. MK-4 is found in animal products, like duck or goose liver (foie gras), some cheeses, and others. Since French people eat plenty of foie gras, maybe this is why they have a lower incidence of heart disease.

MK-7 has become standard of care for prevention of osteoporosis and heart disease because it has a much longer half-life, thus MK-7 only has to be taken once a day, and it is easily detectable in blood analysis. MK-4 has a short half-life of only 1.5 hours and is not detectable in the blood because is quickly taking by the tissues. Much higher doses of MK-4 are required for measurable blood levels, 500 mcg three times daily.

Nevertheless, no clinical study is available comparing MK-4 to MK-7. This opens the door to some experts claiming MK-4 is better because tissues will absorb it quickly. Other experts claim a combination of MK-7 and MK-4 is best. Which vitamin K2 is better, or maybe a combination, is not known at this time. Jeffrey Dach, MD, in *Heart Book* recommends taking both MK-4 and MK-7 but, again, this is not known at this time.

The minimal dose for MK-4 should be 500 mcg three times daily. Osteoporosis has been treated in Japan with 15,000 mcg three times daily (yes, fifteen thousand micrograms three times a day). This dose is available as a supplement in liquid form. [60] A concentrated powder form is also available and is less expensive. [61]

---

60 https://www.thorne.com/products/dp/vitamin-k2-liquid

61 https://superdosing.com/products/vitamin-k2-powder-1000x-1mg-servings-with-scoop?variant=40373016908

In her book *Vitamin K2 and the Calcium Paradox*, Kate Rheaume-Bleue recommends taking 15,000 mcg (15 mg) of vitamin MK-4 three times daily. I think this is more a therapeutic dose (e.g., to reverse coronary calcium or treat osteoporosis) than just prevention.

Unfortunately, the ideal dose for MK-4 has not been established yet. No significant side effects have been reported. There are no contraindications for taking MK-4 in addition to MK-7.

10.1.5. MULTIVITAMIN/MINERALS.

Take one organic multivitamin/mineral pill without iron. Although hemoglobin depends on iron, high levels of iron become toxic quickly. Women in menstrual age might benefit from multivitamins with iron; otherwise, avoid unless you are iron deficient.

Also take ionic minerals because they include all trace minerals the body needs. Take no less than 2.5 ml per day. Dr. Robert Thompson in *The Calcium Lie II* recommends at least 7.5 ml daily.

Avoid colloid minerals. Colloid silver has become popular but I would advise against taking it. Some people take it for the symptomatic relieve of Morgellons disease. Do not. Instead take sodium bicarbonate 5 mg in water twice daily and increase the dose as needed. *Colloidal silver*

10.1.6. OMEGA 3 FATTY ACIDS.

The body needs the omega 3 fatty acids found in fish and other animal products, EPA (eicosapentaenoic acid) and DHA (docosahexaenoic acid). Omega 3 from plants, ALA (alpha-linolenic acid), is poorly converted to the ones used by the body which are EPA and DHA. Although some experts think omega 3 from plants are good enough, most disagree and recommend animal-based omega 3.

Buy a high quality fish oil or cold liver oil of known origin and take 5 to 15 ml daily. Enter your food intake on www.cronometer.com or other similar site to confirm your omega 6:3 ratio is acceptable (1:1 but no greater than 3:1). A larger amount of fish oil can be consumed if trying to decrease inflammation or after strenuous physical activities.

10.1.7. CALCIUM.

Calcium supplements have been shown to have many side effects, including soft tissue calcifications and increased risk of heart attacks, strokes and even all mortality causes. You should get your calcium requirements from food instead until a safe way for taking calcium supplements is found (maybe with vitamin K2). Green leafy vegetables and sesame seeds have good amounts of calcium as well as magnesium.

At least 5 separate studies have demonstrated an increase in coronary heart disease with calcium supplements, ranging from a 15 to 86 percent. Adding vitamin D did not decrease the increased risk of developing heart disease. None of the studies included vitamin K2 (MK-7 or MK-4) in their protocol. Calcium supplements of one gram daily also have been found to increase prostate cancer risk and kidney stones.

If you still decide to take calcium supplements, chose calcium citrate over calcium carbonate and ALWAYS take it with a vitamin K2 MK-7 supplement (at least 90- 120 mcg/day). It would be wise to also add a magnesium supplement. Whether calcium supplements taking with MK-7 and magnesium increase the risk of coronary disease remains to be studied. Until a final answer is available, I would recommend you should meet your calcium requirements by eating a larger amount of green leafy vegetables and organic raw sesame seeds (this calcium is absorbed well) with vitamin D3 supplements if you do not get enough sun exposure.

10.1.8. SUPPLEMENTS TO IMPROVE CELL ENERGY PRODUCTION.

Energy is produced by the mitochondria. If dysfunctional, cells will die or could become cancer cells. Nothing works without enough energy, and cells are no exception.

Improving cell energy production is much more important than taking antioxidants supplements.

A promising supplement to slow down aging is nicotinamide riboside chloride 250 mg daily. Another option is NMN (nicotinamide mononucleotide) 250 gm daily. Although just taking a large dose of niacin might have similar benefits.

In *Mitochondria and the Future of Medicine* Neal Know, ND, recommends several supplements, from what I have selected:

- Resveratrol 1,000 mg daily. It slows down the aging process.
- Pterostilbene 150 mg daily. It works synergistically with resveratrol. They both mimic the benefits of a caloric restricted diet.
- D-Ribose 3-5 gm daily, or a much higher dose might be indicated for certain conditions like fibromyalgia. A 10 to

Mitochondrial NRG

15 g/day has been used in several studies, up to 60 g/day. It is highly recommended for those on a ketogenic diet. D-Ribose is rapidly turned into ATP (energy) by the mitochondria. Although it is a carbohydrate, it does not increase blood sugars. Athletes use D-Ribose before sports to improve their performance and afterwards to recover faster.

- PQD 20 mg daily. PQD stimulates the formation of new mitochondria and can decrease cancer risk.
- Coenzyme Q 10, take 100-300 mg daily. The best absorbed Co Q 10 is a form named Ubiquinol. It increases energy production. One of the several major problems with statin drugs is their interference or reduction of Co Q 10. This has been well known by the pharmaceutical industry for decades. The decrease energy production produces muscle pains, often called "allergic reaction" by medical providers. Knowledgeable medical providers will recommend patients on statins to also take Co Q 10.
- R(+) alpha-lipoic acid has profound anti aging effects, mostly when taken with L-carnitine. 600 mg daily of alpha-lipoic acid (should have at least 300 mg of the R form), store it in the refrigerator.
- L-carnitine 500 mg daily. Available in a bulk (powder) form. Helps production of energy (ATP) by transporting long-chain fatty acids into the mitochondria.
- Magnesium 400 to 1,000 mg/day. Allows the body to use ATP.
- Vitamin B complex. Several vitamin B's are used in energy production.

10.2. SUPPLEMENTS FOR SPECIFIC CONDITIONS

10.2.1. HEART HEALTH

Some heart supplements recommended by Dr. Stephen Sinatra (cardiologist) include:

- Coenzyme Q-10. Take 100 mg of Ubiquinol twice daily.
- D-Ribose 5 grams daily for prevention. 10 to 15 grams daily for heart failure, ischemic cardiovascular disease, or peripheral vascular disease. 15 to 20 grams daily for advanced heart failure and for severe fibromyalgia.
- L-Carnitine 500 mg daily.
- Magnesium supplements, at least 400 mg daily, up to 1,000 mg.

- Niacin decreases LDL and triglycerides with doses of 1,000 mg to 3,000 to 4,000 mg daily. It is one of two major vitamins B3. Avoid the sustained release niacin, it can by hepatotoxic (harm the liver) at relatively low doses. Niacin will increase HDL some, as well as decrease triglycerides. May start with 100 mg after a meal and slowly increase to 500 to 1,000 mg/day. The flushing goes away after some time but recurs with dose increases or if niacin is stopped for a few days. To minimize flushing the first few days, you may take one aspirin before the meal, niacin after the meal.
- Vitamin E with mixed tocopherols 200 IU daily. Some information indicates the tocotrienal forms of vitamin E are better than the tocopherols.
- Omega 3 fatty acids. Take at least one gram daily of EPA and DHA (one gram of DHA for pregnant women) or take high quality fish oil or cold liver oil of known origin.
- Pantethine 300 mg three times daily.
- Consider taking 1 to 2 grams vitamin C daily, curcumin, resveratrol, and cocoa flavonoids (e.g., cocoa powder).

10.2.2. ARTERIOSCLEROSIS/ATHEROSCLEROSIS

Heart disease is reversible. When your physician tells you it is not reversible, what she or he means is prescription medications, e.g. statins, do not decrease arterial calcium/plaques or open up blocked arteries, and this is true. Some patients might not be willing to take appropriate measures to prevent or reverse heart disease. Many others, though, are not aware of what to do. There is some clinical evidence showing heart disease is reversible.

VERY IMPORTANT. *First* stop depositing calcium in your arteries by eating an anti-inflammatory diet, controlling stress, sleeping well, and exercising. The first measure to implement is eating a mostly plant-based organic diet, consuming unheated healthy fats, avoid all refined carbohydrates and man-made fats. Taking supplements or medication without eliminating what is causing the problem to start with does not make any sense and will not be effective.

The two most important supplements to decrease arterial plaque and arterial stiffening are vitamin K2 MK-7 (or MK-4) and magnesium. Vitamin K2 MK-7 is more convenient because it has a longer half-life then MK-4 and, thus, can be taken once daily. At least 90 to 100 mcg/day of MK-7 for adults. 180 to 200 mcg/day is a good dose for adults, at least for prevention. I would favor a higher dose (up to 720 mcg/day) once coronary artery disease, osteoporosis, or other similar condition, has been diagnosed. See vitamin K2 supplement section.

ORAL CHELATION/DETOXIFICATION. The rationale for chronic oral chelation or some type of detoxification is self apparent. We live in a very contaminated planet even though many people are still unaware. For example, on average the amount of lead in our bones is 300 to 500 times greater than before the industrial era. Please remember that no amount of lead in the body is safe.

IV EDTA has been used for advanced coronary artery disease by a few brave pioneer doctors who took the risk of going against the official recommendations. Calcium disodium EDTA should be used (can be given IV in a few minutes and does not rapidly decrease serum calcium), not disodium EDTA. The very expensive national TACT study was sponsored by NCCIH and the National Heart, Lung, and Blood Institute. It showed fewer cardiovascular events in diabetic patients who already had had a heart attack. Unfortunately, the clinical trial used disodium EDTA and did not continue patients on any type of oral protocol. Patients with diabetes benefited from a 41 percent reduction in cardiovascular events, including a 52 percent reduction of another heart attack and a 43 percent reduction in all cause mortality (death rate).

A new ongoing study will try to confirm the indication but no results are available yet. Until then, we will have to wait for a possible FDA approval to treat coronary artery disease. IV disodium EDTA should not be used (takes 3 to 4 hour for the infusion, a severe low blood calcium can happen and a few deaths have been reported). What makes no sense, like it was done in the TACT study, is to treat patients with IV EDTA for a few weeks (e.g., 20 to 30 weekly or biweekly treatments) but then not to continue some type of oral protocol on a chronic basis, that could include or not oral EDTA.

Although EDTA does not actually open blocked arteries, patients have experienced clinical improvement probably because it detoxifies the body from heavy metals like lead and mercury. Those metals are extremely harmful, and there is no known safe level. These metals can oxidize LDL, thus causing heart disease. On a healthy planet people should not have any heavy metals in their bodies but in our case is just the opposite. The amount of heavy metals, like lead, found in our bones is much, much larger than just a few hundred years ago. The generation of electricity with coal plants makes environmental lead contamination worse. Lead from Chinese coal plants has reached other countries, including the USA. What types of not yet commercialized clean energy production technologies could be used is not in the scope of this writing. In the meantime, you are encouraged to chronically detoxify your body.

You could do a screening hair tissue mineral analysis to get an idea how metals might be affecting you. Detoxification protocols should be implemented by everybody on a routine basis.

RECOMMENDATIONS TO DECREASE ARTERIAL PLAQUE.

Of course, do not eat any sugar, refined carbohydrates or bad fats. Avoid heated fats and oils, or at least minimize them and minimize cooking temperatures.

Many natural compounds have anti-plaque properties. Obviously, not all products are needed since there will be a moment when an additional substance will not offer any further improvement. Unfortunately, the ideal combination is not known at this time. The most important supplements are vitamin K2 MK-7 (or MK-4), magnesium, chanca piedra, vitamin D3 (to prevent progression), vitamin C, EDTA, pomegranate, fish omega 3 fatty acids, and Co Q 10.

(A) SPECIFIC RECOMMENDATIONS TO DISSOLVE CALCIUM IN THE ARTERIES.

- Vitamin K2. This supplement is THE MOST IMPORTANT, because it is a supplement that experimentally and clinically has been proven to decrease arterial calcium. Until studies comparing MK-4 to MK-7 become available, it is more convenient taken it as MK-7. This vitamin is in charge of directing calcium to go where it belongs. Thus, it prevents arterial calcium deposits (the ones causing heart attacks) at the same time that improves bone density, thus preventing osteoporosis. It also helps dentition, decreasing dental caries. When a sufficient amount is taking during pregnancy, children develop healthy teeth that do not need orthodontic therapy (braces). Recommended dose in this case is 360 mcg daily, with food because it needs fat for good absorption. Ongoing trials will determine how well can reverse arterial calcium and/or plaque in human beings. Up to 720 mcg per day is a reasonable dose when trying to reverse arterial plaque.
- Magnesium is VERY IMPORTANT also. About 350 enzymes depend on magnesium to work properly, and it is needed for energy (ATP) production. Dose is 400 mg to 1,000 mg daily. You

may need to take it in divided doses to avoid diarrhea. You might need to start with a smaller dose and increase the amount slowly. Chelated magnesium will have less gastrointestinal effects because it has better absorption. Some magnesium supplements are expensive. Magnesium citrate is a good absorption/price compromise.

- Chanca piedra eliminates unwanted calcium deposits. It has also been used for kidney and gallbladder stones. Take 1,000 mg three times daily. It is available bulk in a powder form, as well as pills and liquid. It would be ideal to also take one of the following three supplements. For example, chanca piedra and stone root.

- Stone Root (collinsonia canadensis). Dissolves stone and the arterial system and heart valves. Traditionally, it has been used to dissolve uric acid and calcium stones in the urinary bladder and kidneys. Dose is 1 to 4 grams per day.

- Gravel Root (Eupatorium purpureum). Also called Queen of Meadow. Usually used to treat kidney gravel or stones but helps dissolve calcifications anywhere in the body. It should not be used long-term due to possible hepatoxicity (liver damage). Dose is 1.5 to 2 ml three times daily.

- Hydrangea (Hydrangea arborescens). Mostly used for urinary bladder and kidney gravel and stones but can also be used for the cardiovascular arterial system. Avoid long-term use because no safety studies are available. Dose is 500 to 740 mg once or twice daily

- Organic solutions of hawthorn, garlic, and onion have also been shown to dissolve arterial calcium. Hawthorn in a pill form can be taken as 300 to 600 mg once or twice daily. It seems to be perfectly safe up to 900 mg/day although as much as 1,800 mg daily have been used.

(B) OTHER SUPPLEMENTS TO DISSOLVE CALCIUM IN THE ARTERIES.

- Garlic 2 to 4 fresh cloves daily or fermented garlic. Aged garlic supplements may be used although this option might not be as effective to dissolve calcium but has been found to decrease soft plaque, which is more dangerous than calcified arterial plaque (more heart attacks are due to soft plaque than hard plaque). The dose for aged garlic is 2.4 grams daily (this is the dose used in a study that showed soft plaque regression). Other researchers have used 900 mg/day.

- Pomegranate decreases the narrowing of carotid arteries (carotid stenosis), something statin drugs have failed to accomplish. It also has reversed CAD in mice. Drink a daily glass of pomegranate or, more convenient, take one teaspoon or two of pomegranate powder every day.
- Nattokinase 6,000 FU (600 mg) daily decreased carotid plaque volume by 37 percent, ginger juice diluted in water or mixed with a smoothie 30 ml daily.
- Organic apple cider vinegar diluted in water to dissolve calcium deposits in general. Dose is 10 to 15 ml diluted in water, or other appropriate liquid, twice daily.
- Green algae extract twice daily (like spirulina and chlorella), has decreased carotid plaque by 50 percent.
- Mixed tocotrienols. These are a form of vitamin E which seems to be more effective than mixed tocopherols. Regression of plaque was found in 7 of 25 patients (no regression in the control group). Take 100 mg per day.
- Lemon Essential Oil 10 to 20 drops in a glass of water twice daily. It also helps decrease arterial calcium.

(C) SUPPLEMENTS TO PREVENT FORMATION OR PROGRESSION OF CALCIUM IN THE ARTERIES OR HEART.

- Vitamin D3 has been shown to stop progression of aortic valve calcification. Atherosclerosis is not limited to calcifications and plaque in the coronary (heart) arteries. Arterial calcification happens throughout the circulatory system. One unfortunate location is the aorta. The aortic valve will narrow due to calcium deposits and eventually surgery will be needed. Dr. William Davis (cardiologist) has been able to stop the progression of aortic valve calcification using a therapeutic dose of vitamin D3, on average 8,000 IU per day. This should be done following blood levels of vitamin D3. No regression of the aortic calcification occurred, thus vitamin K2 is still needed. Because vitamin D deficiency increases heart disease risk, vitamin D3 supplements of 4,000 IU to 10,000 IU daily should be taken, ideally checking vitamin D blood levels if the higher dose is taken. Vitamin D serum (blood) levels equal or greater than 75 nmol/L have been found to have protective effect on cardiovascular calcification.

- Oral EDTA. It has not shown to open up blocked arteries but it will decrease the toxic metal load. Several health benefits have been described (see *Detox with Oral Chelation* by David Jay Brown & Gary Gordon, M.D.). Most lead ends up in the bones. To detoxify this lead can take 15 years. How long to remain on oral EDTA, if somebody decided to take it, is beyond the scope of this review. EDTA should be calcium disodium EDTA not sodium EDTA. It is taken on an empty stomach followed by a multi-mineral supplement two hours later. The dose is 1,000 mg daily. Depending on the heavy metal toxic load, the dose can be increased to 1,000 mg twice a day. Let me emphasize a basic concept. I do not think EDTA will remove calcium from the arteries. The main purpose for taking EDTA is to detoxify from the very harmful heavy metals everybody is exposed to. Decreasing the load of heavy metals will improve many health functions, decreasing inflammation in general. EDTA is also available in a sublingual form. EDTA suppositories are available but are more expensive and inconvenient, thus not recommended. In my opinion, the best EDTA is Cardio Renew®, by Cardio Renew Inc., a Minnesota company. It is a liquid form of EDTA with a much higher absorption then traditional pills or powders. No prescription is needed. Initial therapy is fourteen drops in 60 ml of distilled water 5 times daily for six weeks, with at least one hour in between doses. Then, maintenance of 14 drops once daily. Based on price and absorption rate, Cardio Renew® seems to be the best option. It can be purchased on line at https://www.cardiorenew.com/

 Keep homocysteine blood level less than 12 µmol/L by taking TMG (trimethylglycine) 1,500 mg daily. Homocysteine is an independent factor for coronary artery disease. Another way to decrease elevated homocysteine levels is taking supplements of vitamin B6 (10 mg/day), B12 (400 mcg/day), and folic acid (1 mg/day). This combination has been shown to decrease major heart adverse events after percutaneous coronary intervention. [62] Dr. Stephen Sinatra recommends vitamin B6 (5 to 20 mg/day), B12 (400 to 1,000 mcg/day), and folic acid (400 to 800 mcg/day). Plasma folate concentration >39.4 nmol/L has been found to lower homycysteine and prevent arterial calcification.

- Malic acid. It is commercially available in a bulk powder form but often is added to calcium disodium EDTA. The dose is 900 mg once or twice daily. Others use 2 grams daily. It helps detoxification.
- Liposomal vitamin C one gram three times daily. Take it away from meals if you want to minimize iron absorption. Or extended release vitamin C, one gram twice daily.
- N-Acetyl-Cysteine (NAC) at least 200 mg once or twice daily. Or one daily table with 600 mg of NAC with also 50 mcg selenium and 50 mcg molybdenum. It detoxifies metals and pesticides.
- Omega 3 fatty acids. 1 to 2 g/day of omega 3 fish oils (EPA + DHA).
- EGCG 100-200 mg/day, which could be obtained by taking a supplement or by drinking 2 to 5 cups of green tea or 1 to 2 cups of matcha tea daily. EGCG reduces plaque formation.
- R-Lipoic acid 300 mg daily. It lowers the harmful oxidized LDL cholesterol. If you take alpha lipoic acid, then 600 to 1,000 mg/day.
- Co Q 10 200 to 600 mg daily. Ubiquinol is the better form.
- Pueraria Mirifica 50 to 150 mg daily. Traditionally used for menopausal symptoms because it has phytoestrogens.
- Consider strontium 227 to 750 mg/day and boron 3 mg/day supplements, certainly if your hair levels are low. Both help bone health and might help decrease arterial calcium.
- Grape seed extract reduces foam cells. Take 200 mg daily. It is available in a powder form.
- Curcumin 2 to 4 grams daily. Nanocurcumin might be more effective but it is much more expensive.
- Primrose 1,300 mg daily.
- Selenium (as selenomethionine) 200 mcg daily. It helps detoxify mercury and also protects against type 2 diabetes mellitus.

---

62 https://jamanetwork.com/journals/jama/fullarticle/195230

(D) OTHER SUPPLEMENTS THAT CAN HELP DECREASE OR
PREVENT ARTERIAL PLAQUE INCLUDE:

- L-CARNITINE, IMPROVES ENDOTHELIAL FUNCTION.
  DOSE IS 500 MG DAILY. L—Arginine, improves endothelial
  function and increases nitric oxide. Dose is 1,400 to 2,800 mg daily.
- Bergamot 500 mg daily (it also improves carotid arteries).
- Red yeast rice 900 to 1800 mg daily.
- NANOBCTX is a commercially available supplement that
  includes several of the products mentioned above as well as others
  not mentioned but it does not include the very useful vitamin K2
  MK-7, thus you would need to buy it separately.
- Beta cyclodextrin has reversed arterial plaque in vitro and animal
  studies quite well. Unfortunately, it is ototoxic (harms internal ear
  with permanent hearing loss) in humans and, thus, cannot be used
  in clinical practice. Oral alpha cyclodextrin seems to be well
  tolerated and has modestly improved small LDL particles as well
  as improved glucose related parameters.[63]

10.2.3. FOR VEGANS

People on a vegan diet MUST take a vitamin B complex daily. Iron levels
might drop below normal levels on a vegan diet.

10.2.4. HIGH BLOOD PRESSURE (HYPERTENSION)

First, do a mineral hair analysis, called HTMA (hair tissue mineral analysis). [64]
Mineral imbalances and abnormalities should be corrected.

Magnesium 400 to 1,000 mg daily in divided doses. Avoid magnesium
oxide. Take a chelated magnesium for better absorption. Many people with
high blood pressure will see their blood pressures normalize after taking magnesium supplements for several weeks. Magnesium does not decrease a normal
pressure when no magnesium deficiency exists.

Potassium. It is contraindicated in kidney failure. With normal kidney function you could take one teaspoon (5 g) of potassium bicarbonate diluted in
water with a meal daily or even better, 2.5 grams twice a day to avoid irritating
the stomach. Excess potassium can cause diarrhea.

---

63 *Randomized double blind clinical trial on the effect of oral -cyclodextrin on serum lipids.* Amar MJ
et al. Lipids Health Dis. 2016 Jul 12;15(1):115. doi: 10.1186/s12944-016-0284-6.
https://www.ncbi.nlm.nih.gov/pubmed/27405337?dopt=Abstract

64 https://www.doctorsdata.com/hair-elements/

Other supplements are possible but this would be in addition to magnesium and potassium supplements. Hypertension resistant to medications could be secondary to lead intoxication. Most lead is stored in the bones. It has been proposed that post menopausal women sometimes develop high blood pressure when lead is released from the bones while suffering from osteoporosis. This would be an indication to do a hair tissue mineral analysis and heavy metal chelation if indicated.

MORE DETAILED RECOMMENDATIONS:

- Take one capsule of serrapeptase daily (120,000 units-SPU) for at least 6 to 9 months.
- Take one teaspoon (use a measuring teaspoon) of L-Citrulline daily x 6 to 9 months.
- Take one teaspoon (use a measuring teaspoon) of L-Arginine daily x 6 to 9 months.
- Take some type of graviola supplement daily.
- Magnesium. You should be eating 900 mg of elemental magnesium daily. Enter daily food intake into www.cronometer.com to find out how much supplemental magnesium you should take. Magnesium oxide is poorly absorbed so do not take. Use other type of magnesium, like glycinate or orotate. You may take magnesium citrate but be aware it may cause diarrhea, thus take it in divided doses. It might take several weeks or a few months to replenish intracellular magnesium. The ideal ratio of calcium to magnesium intake is 1:1 (current official recommendation says 2:1).
- Potassium. You should be eating 5 g of elemental potassium daily (if no kidney disease/insufficiency). Enter your daily food intake into www.cronometer.com to find out how much supplemental potassium you should take. Best potassium is the one present in foods. Use potassium supplements only if unable to ingest 5 g daily. Potassium bicarbonate powder can be diluted in a glass of water; may add 15 ml of organic apple cider vinegar. It might take several weeks or a few months to replenish intracellular potassium. The ideal ratio of potassium to sodium intake is 2:1.
- Avoid table salt, no exceptions. Use a healthy salt instead. A mostly plant-based diet is ideal and will solve the "salt" problem.

- Avoid processed foods. Non-organic (not free range) chicken often has a large amount of added salt. Do not eat any trans fats (hydrogenated oils) (no exceptions).
- Avoid excess of omega 6 fatty acids (ideal ratio of omega 6 to omega 3 is 1:1), avoid anything greater than 3:1.
- Avoid eating out at restaurants or fast food restaurants.
- Avoid eating the large amount of unhealthy salt that comes with processed food, thus avoid eating processed food. Is best to use Mediterranean, Celtic Sea, or Himalayan salt but use it sparingly initially until your blood pressure normalizes, then you may increase it as tolerated since most people are not "salt sensitive" once they do not have a magnesium and/or potassium deficiency. Sodium bicarbonate (baking soda) does not increase blood pressure because it only has sodium and it is missing the chloride. Rats given intravenous chloride (without sodium) develop high blood pressure.
- Decrease your weight to a normal BMI (< 25) (percentage of body fat is more accurate but more cumbersome to measure) or as close to normal as possible. For practical instructions, see the books *Fat For Fuel* by Dr. Joseph Mercola and *How Not To Diet* by Dr. Michael Gregger.
- Avoid sleep deprivation or changes in circadian sleep cycles (e.g., always sleep the same time of day, ideally at night to benefit from sun light)
- Control stress. Meditation is ideal, as described elsewhere.
- Exercise regularly (HIIT is the best exercise).

10.2.5. WEIGHT LOSS

Several supplements have been recommended in combination for weight loss but not a single supplement works well. The Z plan diet, though, provides a spray that seems to work well controlling hunger cravings.

10.2.6. CATARACTS

Detoxify.

Can C (N-Acetylcarnosine) eye drops twice daily for a few months. For advanced cataracts, you will need surgery.

10.2.7. OSTEOPOROSIS

Avoid calcium supplements or food fortified with calcium because studies have shown to increase the risk of heart disease. You should get your calcium needs from food and the healthiest sources are green leafy vegetables and raw sesame seeds. Calcium needs magnesium to prevent osteoporosis, in addition to other minerals and trace minerals. Some experts recommend a 1:1 ration of calcium:magnesium. Vitamin D added to calcium supplements has not been able to eliminate or reduce the increased risk of heart disease. Whether calcium supplements taking in conjunction with vitamin K2 MK-7 (or K2 MK-4) could benefit bone density without increasing the risk of heart disease is not known at this time. Just in case, my advice is to avoid calcium supplements or foods fortified with calcium.

- Vitamin K2. Most experts think it should be MK-7 because it has a longer half-life then MK-4. At least 90 to 100 mcg/day. Even 180 mcg/day is a safe and a good dose for prevention in adults. It should be taking in conjunction with vitamin D (4,000 or 5,000 IU daily) and magnesium supplements (400 to 1,000 mg/day). Whether taking additional MK-4 could provide extra benefits is not known. A higher dose of MK-4 (up to 1,500 mcg three times daily) is needed and it should be taken three times daily due to its short half life. For somebody with osteoporosis or for post menopausal women, take at least 240 mcg daily of MK-7 (or 1,500 mcg of MK-4 three times daily).
- Vitamin D3. 4,000 or 5,000 IU daily is safe. Up to 10,000 IU daily is probably safe. If the latter amount is taking for months or years, or if taking a higher dose, follow your vitamin D blood levels to make sure you are not getting into toxic levels. Vitamin D toxicity can cause hypercalcemia (increased calcium in the blood) and other complications.
- Magnesium supplements 400 to 1,000 mg/day for most people.
- Silica is a micronutrient needed for healthy bone. 325 mcg (2 ml) of liquid silicon dioxide for a few days will probably meet the body requirements.
- Balanced ionic trace minerals daily. Robert Thompson, MD and Kathleen Barnes in The Calcium Lie II recommend 3 grams daily of essential balanced trace minerals, or one and a half

teaspoon (7.5 ml) of the liquid form. Also, do a mineral hair analysis and replace any deficient minerals, specifically sodium, magnesium, and potassium. Do not take any colloid minerals, not even to replace a deficiency. Based on Dr. Thompson, 90 percent of people might be deficient in intra-cellular sodium. Avoid bromine or foods with bromine because it is a mineral disrupter. Avoid toxic levels of any mineral as they can interfere with others. Dr. Thompson recommends using chelated minerals only for the short term replacement of a mineral deficiency. Other authors recommend taking chelated minerals on a chronic basis, like magnesium malate (see Calcification: The Aging Factor by Mark Mayer).

Never use table salt because it is processed in an unhealthy way and is depleted from other necessary minerals. Only use healthy salts, like Mediterranean, Celtic Sea, or Himalayan salts because they have trace minerals needed by the bones to maintain normal density.

Weight-bearing exercises, of course, are a must in addition to supplements.

10.2.8. ERECTILE DYSFUNCTION
- Amino acids combination. Arginine 2.5-5 g daily and citrulline 2.5 g daily. Both are available in bulk powder form. They increase the production of nitric oxide which relaxes vessels thus improving circulation.
- DHEA if testosterone levels are low. Dose is 100 mg daily.
- Pycnogenol 100 mg twice daily.
- Consider shock wave therapy. Most clinical studies have found it to be successful and has no side effects. Of course, you must eat a healthy non-inflammatory diet.

10.2.9. FIBROMYALGIA
- D-Ribose, start with 5 to 10 grams daily and increase as needed.
- Vitamin D to keep vitamin D levels on the high side.
- Magnesium 1,000 mg daily in several divided doses. Magnesium malate is a good choice.
- Malic acid 1200 to 2400 mg daily.
- Consider intense detoxification and eliminate all environmental toxins.

- Restore gut health with probiotics and avoiding unhealthy foods (like GMO food, foods with glyphosate, and NSAIDS).

10.2.10. ATRIAL FIBRILLATION
- Magnesium 400 to 1,000 mg daily for several weeks to restore intracellular storages. Ionic trace minerals daily.

11. STUDIES

11.1. LABORATORY STUDIES (SEROLOGY/BLOOD).

11.1.1. HIGH SENSITIVE CRP.
It detects inflammation. In the absence of acute inflammation, indicates chronic inflammation. Ideally, it should be under 1 (other experts say under 0.8). If higher, additional work up and intervention is needed. As mentioned above, predicts heart attacks better then total cholesterol and LDL.

11.1.2. FASTING GLUCOSE (AT LEAST 8 HOURS WITHOUT ANY FOOD INTAKE).
Normal is under 100 but ideal is 86 or less. The higher the worse, 126 or higher being diabetes (should repeat measurement more than once) and between 100 and 125 is considered prediabetes although it would preferable to do a hemoglobin A1c.

11.1.3. TWO HOUR POST MEAL GLUCOSE.
It should be under 140 but ideal is under 120. A better idea of how a meal is affecting glucose is to measure at 1, 2, and 3 hours after a meal in the comfort of your home. If the 3-hour glucose is higher than the 2-hour one, continue every hour until blood glucose starts decreasing. A 3-hour blood glucose significantly higher than the 2-hour one indicates the fat ingested is blocking the insulin receptor, thus avoid that food product.

11.1.4. A1C HEMOGLOBIN.
There is no need to fast for this test. It is available over the counter or by mail order. It measures the three prior month blood glucose average. Half of its value is determined by the last thirty days. The lower the better although it has a small J curve (worse prognosis when it is very low, which is usually under 5). Normal is 4.5 to 5.6. Prediabetes is 5.7 to 6.4. Diabetes can be diagnosed

once it reaches 6.5. The higher over 6.5, the worse is the diabetic control. Worse diabetic control implies many more diabetic complications. In some studies diabetic complications were not reduced despite glucose control but this is probably because some diabetes medications increase insulin production and this has long term side effects (increased insulin levels are pro-inflammatory). Other medications that do not increase insulin levels (like Metformin) should decrease long term complications. A healthy plant-based diet, eco ketogenic or at least low in carbohydrates, and making sure you do not eat any refined carbohydrates should improve the outcome of patients with diabetes. Check A1c as frequently as indicated for your condition or to find out how you are responding to a diet, like a plant-based diet or an eco ketogenic diet.

11.1.5. FASTING INSULIN.

Low blood fasting insulin levels correlate well with longer survival. This test is not routinely done by primary care providers and you will have to request it. It will provide you with years of advance notice of a brewing medical condition. It will be much easier to prevent type 2 diabetes if you correct an elevated fasting insulin now than if you wait until you have developed prediabetes or diabetes. If you are not able to lose weight as expected, make sure your fasting insulin is low (less than 3 or 5 depending on the expert). Some experts also recommend a 2-hour post meal blood insulin level but I would delegate to your expert provider to decide whether this test would benefit you.

11.1.6. FERRITIN.

A high ferritin significantly increases the risk of heart attacks. This is the reason menstruating women have less heart attacks unless they undergo an early hysterectomy. Women's risk of heart disease increases in a parallel line to men after they reach menopause. Two studies showed hormonal replacement (estrogens) after menopause did not decrease heart disease but increased breast cancers. A lower ferritin/iron level is also why blood donation (at least once per year) decreases the risk of heart attacks. If you have any medical contraindications to blood donation, you still can request a medical flebotomy (your blood will be withdrawn but discarded).

11.1.7. LIPID PANEL.

A traditional lipid panel is routinely ordered by medical providers. Total cholesterol and LDL (which are often used to decide whether to start a statin medication) are not good predictors of heart disease. High triglycerides (TG) are more reliable. They should be under 150 but ideal is under 100. High tri-glycerides increase the risk of heart disease and are usually due to overconsumption of carbohydrates or to trans fats. Eliminate all refined car-bohydrates (e.g., flour, bread, pasta, pizza, etc.), decrease other carbohydrates, do not eat any bad fats, and your triglycerides will greatly improve.

The higher the HDL the better. The triglyceride/HDL ratio is a good in-direct way to estimate how much bad LDL is present (the oxidized small dense particles). Ideal TG/HDL ratio should be under 2. If it is higher, you could ask your provider to perform a LDL particle blood test, which will be a much better prognostic indicator than total cholesterol and/or calculated LDL. Commercially available LDL particle tests include NMR test, the Lipoprotein Particle Profile test (LPP), the Berkeley cholesterol test, and the Verticle Auto Profile test (VAP). Just one will suffice.

11.1.8. OTHER STUDIES SHOULD BE BASED ON PERSONAL FACTORS (E.G., RULE OUT HYPOTHYROIDISM IF UNABLE TO LOSE WEIGHT, RULE OUT METAL POISONING, ETC.)

11.2. CARDIAC SCAN

A cardiac scan can be used to assess coronary artery disease risk and to deter-mine therapeutic efficacy, i.e. whether therapeutic measures implemented have been successful or not. It is also called a coronary calcium study or score. It is a CT scan of the chest that measures the amount of calcium in the cor-onary arteries. Normal is 0 (no calcium), minimal is under ten, mild is 10 to 99, moderate is 100 to 399, severe is 400 to 999, and extensive is 1,000 or higher. This amount of calcium correlates with the degree of heart disease and risk for future heart attacks. In addition, coronary artery calcium (CAC) "is also strongly associated with the development of stroke and congestive heart failure." Data has shown "worse prognosis associated with increasing CAC (coronary artery calcium) on serial scans" which means it can be used not just to evaluate heart disease risk but also to determine how successful a therapeutic intervention was. [65]

A cardiac scan has been found to be "one of the strongest individual tests for determining long-term ASCVD (atherosclerotic cardiovascular disease) risk in an asymptomatic patient." [66]

---

65 *Coronary Artery Calcium Scanning Past, Present, and Future.* Hecht HS. J Am Coll Cardiol Img 2015: 8:579-96. http://imaging.onlinejacc.org/content/jimg/8/5/579.full.pdf.

66 *CAC-DRS: Coronary Artery Calcium Data and Reporting System. An expert consensus document of*

A multivariable analysis in the MESA study showed that the only predictive variable was a cardiac scan score greater than 100. [67]

The purpose of the study is to detect coronary disease early on so that life style changes, some supplements (like vitamin K2 MK-7, etc.), and dietary changes can be implemented.

When to perform this test is controversial because it delivers a small amount of radiation. Despite all the scientific evidence available, usually a cardiac scan is not covered by insurance companies, which seem to be focusing on treatment more than prevention. Nevertheless, it can be paid pre-tax with a health savings account and large medical institutions charge about $100. Doing at least a baseline study seems reasonable for some people. It would not be indicated if a diagnosis of coronary artery disease has already been made. For asymptomatic men with low risk for cardiac disease, maybe age 60 is a good age, but could be done several years earlier for those with a significant family history of heart attacks or other major risk factors. In women, at or after age 65 if they do not have any risk factors. But, again, there is no good consensus on this advice.

The Society of Cardiovascular Computed Tomography recommendation is "It is appropriate to perform CAC testing in the context of shared decision making for asymptomatic individuals without clinical ASCVD who are 40–75 years of age in the 5–20 percent 10-year ASCVD risk group and selectively in the <5 percent ASCVD group, such as those with a family history of premature coronary artery disease." (CAC = coronary artery calcium. ASCVD = atherosclerosis cardiovascular disease) [68]

the *Society of Cardiovascular Computed Tomography (SCCT)*. Hecht HS, et al. Journal of Cardiovascular Computed Tomography, 2018-05-01, Volume 12, Issue 3, Pages 185-191. https://www.clinicalkey.com/#!/content/playContent/1-s2.0-S1934592518300583?returnurl=https:%2F%2Flinkinghub.elsevier.com%2Fretriev e%2Fpii%2FS1934592518300583%3Fshowall%3Dtrue&referrer=https:%2F%2Fw ww.ncbi.nlm.nih.gov%2Fpubmed%2F29793848

67 *Coronary artery Calcium predicts Cardiovascular events in participants with a low lifetime risk of Cardiovascular disease: The Multi-Ethnic Study of Atherosclerosis (MESA). Joshi PH, et al. Atherosclerosis.* 2016 Mar;246:367-73. doi: 10.1016/j.atherosclerosis.2016.01.017. Epub 2016 Jan 13. https://www.ncbi.nlm.nih.gov/pubmed/26841074

68 Clinical indications for coronary artery calcium scoring in asymptomatic patients: Expert consensus statement from the Society of Cardiovascular Computed Tomography. Hecht H, et al. Journal of Cardiovascular Computed Tomography, 2017-03-01, Volume 11, Issue 2, Pages 157-168. https://www.clinicalkey.com/#!/content/playContent/1-s2.0-S1934592517300461?returnurl=https:%2F%2Flinkinghub.elsevier.com%2Fretrieve%2F pii%2FS1934592517300461%3Fshowall%3Dtrue&referrer=https:%2F%2Fwww.ncbi.nl m.nih.gov%2Fpubmed%2F28283309

If the study is normal (no calcium, score = 0), it is good for 5 years. In can be repeated in 3 to 5 years if it is abnormal although some clinicians might recommend it sooner to evaluate how successful therapeutic interventions were.

You may read more information at:

https://www.sciencedirect.com/science/article/pii/S1936878X15001369

https://ac.els-cdn.com/S1936878X15001369/1-s2.0-S1936878X15001369-main.pdf?tid=50c4503d-b396-4bdd-9f17-45f7e7f63280&acdnat=155537 8018140897c0e36865aef6c4c0e3a7918e73

11.3. HAIR ANALYSIS (HTMA – HAIR TISSUE MINERAL ANALYSIS)

Our planet is very polluted, much worse that what most people realize. It all started with the industrial revolution and there is no light at the end of the tunnel. A small hair sample allows for testing of heavy metals and minerals in the comfort of your home. Both toxic levels and deficiencies can be found. Consult with the appropriate medical provider if you have any significant abnormal findings. This testing can be ordered online, and the results will be available a few days after mailing the hair samples. It is reasonable to at least do a one-time screening analysis, at least for heavy metals. High levels of lead, mercury, cadmium, etc. have major long-term side effects. If toxic levels are found, consult with a specialist. This also can be done online.

In addition, hair analysis can be used for nutritional deficiencies and sensitivities. [69] As an example, a lithium deficiency can cause mood problems and irritability. It cannot be detected with a blood test but a hair analysis will diagnose it.

I have done several hair analyses, to family members and myself, using *Doctor's Data Essential Elements and Heavy Metals Toxicity Test*, which can be purchased online without a doctor's order. In my experience, this test is very reliable.

11.4. BONE DENSITY SCAN

At age 65 both for men and women. It might need to be done at an earlier age based on risk factors, like cigarette smoking, low physical activity, etc.

12. FUNCTIONAL MEDICINE

Functional or integrative medicine providers should be able to assist with the management of intoxication by heavy metals, food allergies and sensitivities, and nutritional deficiencies. Stool studies can be done to rule out a leaky gut.

---

69 https://smile.amazon.com/gp/product/B01J6RZTLC/ref=ppxyodtbasintitleo0 4s01?ie=UTF8&psc=1

13. DOCUMENTARIES

Some good food documentaries available on Netflix include *Hungry for Change; Forks over Knives; Food Matters; PlantPure Nation; Sugar Coated; Fed Up; Fat, Sick, and Nearly Dead* (1 and 2); *GMO OMG; Food, Inc.; Cowspiracy; Food Choices; In Defense of Food;* and *What the Health.* Available on YouTube are Dr. Robert Lustig's videos *Sugar: The Bitter Truth; Fat Chance: Fructose 2.0* and *Is a calorie a calorie Processed Food, Experiment Gone Wrong.* Documentaries about vaccines (not available on Netflix) include *For the Greater Good, Bought,* and *Vaxxed* among several others.

14. OTHER REFERENCES:

1.14.1. CANCER AND SODIUM BICARBONATE (BAKING SODA).

- http://www.ncbi.nlm.nih.gov/pubmed/25376898 Cancer Metastasis Rev. 2014 Dec;33(4):1095-108. doi: 10.1007/s10555-014-9531-3. Microenvironmental acidosis in carcinogenesis and metastases: new strategies in prevention and therapy.
- http://www.ncbi.nlm.nih.gov/pubmed/25102038 J Pain Palliat Care Pharmacother. 2014 Sep; 28(3):206-11. doi: 10.3109/15360288.2014.938882. Epub 2014 Aug 7. Palliative treatment for advanced biliary adenocarcinomas with combination dimethyl sulfoxide-sodium bicarbonate infusion and S-adenosyl-L-methionine.
- http://www.ncbi.nlm.nih.gov/pubmed?term=Investigating%20mec hanisms%20of%20al kalinization%5BTitle%5D Biomed Res Int.; 2013:485196. doi: 10.1155/2013/485196. Epub 2013 Jul 10. Investigating mechanisms of alkalinization for reducing primary breast tumor invasion.
- http://www.ncbi.nlm.nih.gov/pubmed/19276390 Cancer Res. 2009 Mar 15;69(6):2260-8. doi: 10.1158/0008-5472.CAN-07-5575. Epub 2009 Mar 10. Bicarbonate increases tumor pH and inhibits spontaneous metastases.
- http://www.ncbi.nlm.nih.gov/pubmed/21861189 Clin Exp Metastasis. 2011 Dec;28(8):841-9. doi: 10.1007/s10585-011-9415-7. Epub 2011 Aug 23. Reduction of metastasis using a non-volatile buffer.

1.14.2. EARTHING OR GROUNDING.

- https://heartmdinstitute.com/alternative-medicine/earthing/what-is-earthing-or-grounding/
- http://www.ncbi.nlm.nih.gov/pubmed/18047442 J Altern Complement Med. 2007 Nov;13(9):955-67. Can electrons act as antioxidants? A review and commentary.
- http://www.ncbi.nlm.nih.gov/pubmed/25848315 J Inflamm Res. 2015 Mar 24;8:83-96. doi: 10.2147/JIR.S69656. eCollection 2015.The effects of grounding (earthing) on inflammation, the immune response, wound healing, and prevention and treatment of chronic inflammatory and autoimmune diseases.
- http://www.ncbi.nlm.nih.gov/pubmed/15650465 J Altern Complement Med. 2004 Oct;10(5):767-76. The biologic effects of grounding the human body during sleep as measured by cortisol levels and subjective reporting of sleep, pain, and stress.
- http://www.ncbi.nlm.nih.gov/pubmed/25748085 Psychol Rep. 2015 Apr;116(2):534- 42. doi: 10.2466/06.PR0.116k21w5. Epub 2015 Mar 6. The effect of grounding the human body on mood.
- http://www.ncbi.nlm.nih.gov/pubmed/20192911 J Altern Complement Med. 2010 Mar;16(3):265-73. doi: 10.1089/acm.2009.0399. Pilot study on the effect of grounding on delayed-onset muscle soreness.
- http://www.ncbi.nlm.nih.gov/pubmed/21856083 Med Hypotheses. 2011 Nov;77(5):824-6. doi: 10.1016/j.mehy.2011.07.046. The neuromodulative role of earthing.
- http://www.ncbi.nlm.nih.gov/pubmed/22420736 J Altern Complement Med. 2012 Mar;18(3):229-34. doi: 10.1089/acm.2010.0683. Earthing the human organism influences bioelectrical processes.
- http://www.ncbi.nlm.nih.gov/pubmed/22757749 J Altern Complement Med. 2013 Feb;19(2):102-10. doi: 10.1089/acm.2011.0820. Epub 2012 Jul 3. Earthing (grounding) the human body reduces blood viscosity-a major factor in cardiovascular disease.
- http://www.ncbi.nlm.nih.gov/pubmed/22291721 J Environ Public Health. 2012;2012:291541. doi: 10.1155/2012/291541. Epub 2012

Jan 12. *Earthing: health implications of reconnecting the human body to the Earth's surface electrons.*

- http://www.ncbi.nlm.nih.gov/pubmed/21469913 J Altern Complement Med. 2011 Apr;17(4):301-8. doi: 10.1089/acm.2010.0687. Epub 2011 Apr 6. Earthing the human body influences physiologic processes.
- http://www.ncbi.nlm.nih.gov/pubmed/25376898 Cancer Metastasis Rev. 2014 Dec;33(4):1095-108. doi: 10.1007/s10555-014-9531-3. Microenvironmental acidosis in carcinogenesis and metastases: new strategies in prevention and therapy.
- http://www.ncbi.nlm.nih.gov/pmc/articles/PMC3265077/ J Environ Public Health. 2012; 2012: 291541. Published online 2012 Jan 12. doi: 10.1155/2012/291541 PMCID: PMC3265077 Earthing: Health Implications of Reconnecting the Human Body to the Earth's Surface Electrons.
- http://www.ncbi.nlm.nih.gov/pmc/articles/PMC4378297/ J Inflamm Res. 2015; 8: 83-96. The effects of grounding (earthing) on inflammation, the immune response, wound healing, and prevention and treatment of chronic inflammatory and autoimmune diseases.
- Published online 2015 Mar 24. doi: 10.2147/JIR.S69656 PMCID: PMC4378297. The effects of grounding (earthing) on inflammation, the immune response, wound healing, and prevention and treatment of chronic inflammatory and autoimmune diseases.
- Earthing. The most important health discovery ever! By Clinton Ober, Stephen T. Sinatra, M.D., and Marin Zucker.

1.14.3. BLOOD DONATION.

- http://jnci.oxfordjournals.org/content/100/14/996.abstract JNCI: Jnl of National Cancer Institute 2008; Volume 100, Issue 14 Pp. 996-1002. Decreased Cancer Risk After Iron Reduction in Patients With Peripheral Arterial Disease: Results From a Randomized Trial.
- http://aje.oxfordjournals.org/content/148/5/445.full.pdf Am J Epidemiol 1998; 148 (5): 445-51. Donation of Blood Is Associated with Reduced Risk of Myocardial Infarction The Kuopio Ischaemic Heart Disease Risk Factor Study.

- http://www.medicaldaily.com/why-donating-blood-good-your-health-246379
- https://www.organicfacts.net/health-benefits/other/blood-donation.html
- http://www.rasmussen.edu/degrees/health-sciences/blog/surprising-health-benefits-of-donating-blood/

15. ALTERNATIVE NON-TRADITIONAL THERAPIES FOR CANCER TREATMENT AND OTHER DISEASES

These are therapies not recognized by the current "standard of care" consensus. Readers should do their own research.

15.1. GCMAF

GcMAF stands for Gc protein-derived macrophage activating factor and is a protein that stimulates the immune system. See https://gcmaf.se/how-gcmaf-works/ for a detailed explanation. Reputable physicians, like Dr. Russell Blaylock in his Wellness Report, have stated GcMAF has been successful treating a variety of cancers. This therapy is commercially available. Visit https://gcmaf.se/

15.2. CHLORINE DIOXIDE THERAPY

Chlorine dioxide therapy is not part of the armamentarium of official medicine although it is commercially available and it is used by some municipalities for city water treatment and disinfection. Dioxide is different than chlorine which is also used for water purification.

Some people know it as MMS, a term coined by Jim Humble, who has published several books on this subject. The books can be purchased from his website since other retailers are blocking their sale. MMS initially meant miracle mineral solution but Jim Humble now calls it master mineral solution, instead. It has been used for the treatment of malaria. Jim Humble has protocols for multiple medical conditions. Chlorine dioxide (CD) is very soluble in water. It is made my mixing same amounts of 24% sodium chlorite 4% hydrochloric acid, waiting about one minute, and then mixing 24 drops with one liter of distilled or mineral water. Then, the person drinks the resulting solution every hour over an eight hour period. Alternatively, it is acceptable mixing 28 percent sodium chlorite with 5 percent hydrochloric acid.

A better option, probably, is using chlorine dioxide solution (CDS) because it is pH neutral and, thus, it does not cause any gastrointestinal symptoms, like stomach irritation or diarrhea. Ample information is available on how to make it, which can be easily accomplished at home. The final solution will have 3,000 PPM (parts per million) of chlorine dioxide. I find easier to make a 1,500 PPM solution but use twice the amount a treatment protocol calls for. The initial starting dose is 10 milliliters of the 3,000 PPM solution added to one liter of distilled or mineral water. The maximum dose is eight times this amount. One hundred milliliters of the diluted mixture are ingested every hour, for a total of 10 hours. As a general detoxification protocol, this can be done daily for 3 to 6 weeks. Chlorine dioxide solution is also commercially available, although is only advertised for non-medical uses and it is more expensive than making it at home. https://waterpureworld.com/

Chlorine dioxide therapy has been used for cancer treatment but also for many other diseases, too numerous to enumerate here. A detailed explanation with several protocols is available in the book *Forbidden Health: Incurable Was Yesterday* by Andreas Ludwig Kalcker. The original book in Spanish was published in Spain but it has been translated to several languages, including English. Major distributers are censoring this book, blocking its sale, but it can be purchased directly from the publisher at https://voedia.com/en/

I estimated the cost of one month treatment using commercially available sodium chlorite and hydrochloric acid to be as low as $1.6 (using 10 ml of homemade chlorine dioxide solution in one liter of water daily).

I have seen good results with this treatment for several non-cancer conditions. Acute viral infections (common cold) seem to respond well to the "Frequent" protocol described by Kalcker. I have personally experienced a significant improvement in fasting blood glucose (from normal to lower normal blood sugars), although this improvement took at least 2 to 3 months and was more pronounced with a higher dose (30 ml of CDS instead of the starting 10 ml dose).

15.3. HULDA REGEHR CLARK'S, PH.D, TREATMENT PROTOCOL FOR CANCER

Dr. Clark spent many decades studying the cause and treatment of all cancers. My advice is to follow the standard of care for cancer therapy. Nevertheless, for those with "incurable" cancers that are beyond the knowledge of current medical therapy, it would reasonable to at least read the treatments she describes in her book The Cure and Prevention of All Cancers. I do not know how successful her therapy will be but what does a person with an incurable or terminal cancer have to lose? She recommends an extensive protocol, too complex to describe here.

15.4. KETOGENIC DIET WITH GLUTAMINE INHIBITORS

Cancer cells are anaerobic, which means they must use a very large amount of glucose to survive. The basic concept is starving cancer cells by eating a very low carbohydrate diet. In reality the mechanism is not that simple since cancer cells also utilize fructose and glutamine. This diet has been used with some success and is being studied in some major cancer centers as an additional therapy.

Several herbs have been used to prevent cancer cells from using glutamine, which cancer cells can get from muscle cells. EGCG (epigallocatechin-3-gallate) has been used as a glutamine inhibitor. It can be found in matcha and green teas. One tablespoon of matcha tea (about 2.5 g) has 125 mg of EGCG.

A ketogenic diet with glutamine inhibitors has been used by Dr. Thomas Seyfried, a professor of biology at Boston College in Chestnut Hill, Massachusetts.

More information on a ketogenic diet is available in the book *The Metabolic Approach to Cancer* by Dr. Nasha Winters, ND, L.Ac., FABNO, and Jess Higgins Kelly, MNT.

15.5. FENBENDAZOLE

Fenbendazole is an animal antiparasitic medication. It has been found to have anticancer properties.[70] This medication is very inexpensive, thus the pharmaceutical industry does not have a financial interest to promote it. Joe Tippens was diagnosed with terminal metastatic small cell lung cancer. A PET scan confirmed his cancer had spread widely. For "modern medicine", this is an incurable cancer. Joe took febendazole in addition to curcumin and CBD (cannabis oil) and his cancer completely melted away. Joe is testing this therapy, so far in about one hundred patients. For more information you may watch YouTube https://www.youtube.com/watch?v=-WxiPf-NEDk or visit his webpage https://www.mycancerstory.rocks/

Further useful information can be found at https://thetruthabout cancer.com/category/cancer-treatments/

15.6. DCA THERAPY

Dichloroacetate (DCA) is used in Canadian clinics for the treatment of cancer patients (https://medicorcancer.com/). The goal is to stabilize the disease. The rationale for using DCA is available at https://medicorcancer.com/dca-therapy/

---

70 http://ar.iiarjournals.org/content/33/2/355.full *(Fenbendazole as a Potential Anticancer Drug)*.

15.7. VITAMIN B17

Vitamin B17 contains cyanide. Cancer cells have an enzyme, beta-glucosidase, that releases the cyanide. Normal cells do not have this enzyme. In addition, normal cells but not cancer cells have rhodanese, a cyanide-neutralizing enzyme.

Vitamin B17 is not commercially available in the USA but can be obtained by buying raw bitter apricot seeds. It must be bitter seeds since non-bitter apricot seeds do not contain cyanide. Bitter almonds also have vitamin B17 but are difficult, if not impossible, to find because farmers have eliminated them from their crops.

For prevention, use 5 to 10 organic raw bitter apricot kernels. For therapy a significantly larger dose has been used by some. A word of caution, though— the dose should be increased slowly to decrease the risk of cyanide poisoning.

A detailed history of vitamin B17 can be found in *World without Cancer. The story of Vitamin B17* by G. Edward Griffin.

15.8. SODIUM BICARBONATE.

Sodium bicarbonate is baking soda. No prescription is needed. Do not confuse with baking powder. Baking soda is very inexpensive and is quite effective in preventing most cancers because it increases the body's pH. Most cancers need an acidic environment for proper growth and propagation. Some cancers are not pH dependent, though, like melanomas.

For prevention, 5 g (one teaspoon) diluted in a glass of water once or twice a day will suffice. This small dose might also decrease cancer metastases (cancer spread). As a therapy for cancer, much higher doses have been proposed. 0.5 g/Kg/day have been used.[71]

I doubt sodium bicarbonate will be useful as a therapeutic agent, at least if used alone. Once a cancer is well established, it creates its own acidic environment and sodium bicarbonate will not be able to reach or neutralize it.

15.9. FIVE-DAY FAST

A 5-day fast or a 5-day mimicking diet as described by Valter Longo, Ph.D., in his book *The Longevity Diet*. Fasting did not kill cancer cells but improved the effects of chemotherapy in Dr. Longo's clinical trials.

Fasting will increase autophagy (the recycling of old organelles within the cells) and this should prevent or decrease cancers in general. This is another example of preventive measures being superior to therapeutic intervention.

---

71 https://clinicaltrials.gov/ct2/show/NCT02531919

15.10. ELECTROMAGNETIC FREQUENCY THERAPY

Electromagnetic frequency therapy induces scalar or transverse waves which are not acknowledge by modern medicine and, thus, have not been well studied. This technology is being used to treat many different diseases including acute viral infections. It has the potential to benefit cancer patients but clinical trials are not available.

Several devices are commercially available. Biotrohn by Medalab Technologies is the most advanced device. It is manufactured in Spain and available to the public. It can be purchased directly from the manufacturer at http://biotrohn.net/ This technology has been endorsed by the European Union.